Participation in Children and Young People's Mental Health

Participation in Children and Young People's Mental Health: An Essential Guide aims to break down the historical challenges surrounding children and young people's mental health (CYPMH) participation.

It explores topics from how to conceptualise participation to more practical advice and guidance surrounding how to 'do' participation. Uniquely edited by Experts-by-Experience, it offers useful insights into how participation ought to be led from those with experience in the field. This ground-breaking text is supported by contributions from leading experts, including a mixture of lived experience and academic perspectives, providing a comprehensive dive into key concepts and practical examples to help improve practice. The chapters aim to spark thinking, conversations, and actions relating to participation and will provide lessons to embed it into services, organisations, areas, groups, practice, and work.

This text is an essential guide for trainees and professionals working in CYPMH services which includes the NHS in England, the voluntary sector, and other health systems internationally.

Hannah Sharp is an international consultant on patient participation in children and young people's mental health services. She holds a Bachelor's degree in Social and Political Sciences with Philosophy.

Leanne Walker has worked for the last decade locally, nationally, and internationally in the mental health lived experienced field and has a postgraduate certificate in transformational leadership.

Participation in Children and Young People's Mental Health

An Essential Guide

Edited by
Hannah Sharp and Leanne Walker

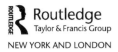

Routledge
Taylor & Francis Group

NEW YORK AND LONDON

Designed cover image: Leanne Walker

First published 2024
by Routledge
605 Third Avenue, New York, NY 10158

and by Routledge
4 Park Square, Milton Park, Abingdon, Oxon OX14 4RN

Routledge is an imprint of the Taylor & Francis Group, an informa business

Library of Congress Cataloging-in-Publication Data
A catalog record for this title has been requested

ISBN: 978-1-032-26552-0 (hbk)
ISBN: 978-1-032-26551-3 (pbk)
ISBN: 978-1-003-28880-0 (ebk)

DOI: 10.4324/9781003288800

Typeset in Times New Roman
by Taylor & Francis Books

To all living with or who have lived with mental health difficulties, and everyone supporting people through it, we see you and this book is for you.

Contents

Illustrations

Figures

Table

Contributors

Yvonne Anderson specialises in co-production with children and young people. She worked as part of the team driving the patient participation element of the Children and Young People's Improving Access to Psychological Therapies programme and has extensive knowledge of how we engage children and young people in national policy, service development, and their own care.

Nikki Chapman, an adoptive parent, and former foster carer has lived experience of supporting children with mental health difficulties. She is the co-founder of the Fresh Plus Group working in partnership with Alder Hey Children's NHS Foundation Trust, co-lead of the Rethinking Education: Lessons from Lockdown Special Interest Research Group and a member of the Emerging Minds Advisory Board. She's also a member of the PLACE Network which aims to develop, promote, and sustain parent and carer support and involvement in mental health across the UK. As an expert by experience, she delivers training on parent participation across the Northwest.

Amanda Cooper has worked in the mental health sector since the age of 16. She has commented on various documents for NICE, The Children's Mental Health Taskforce, the Health Select Committee and MILESTONE, an EU funded pan-European research project, to which she has works co-authored published by Lancet psychiatry. She was a co-chair of the service development group which steered national service transformation through the Children and Young People's Improving Access to Psychological Therapies programme. Amanda was also an ambassador for the Time to Change charity tackling stigma and discrimination of mental health illnesses. Amanda now 30, currently resides in South Yorkshire with her daughter and husband and is hoping to start a new career in midwifery in the near future.

Ann Cox is a CAMHS nurse consultant and is an honorary senior lecturer at Keele University. She passionately works closely with children, young people, and their families as part of their own care. She holds a doctorate in health and social care practice (nursing) where she focused her work on how younger children can be better involved in their care ethically and safely.

Amari Creak is a children and young people's mental health advocate. They work as a lived experience partner for NHS England, a peer consultant for the mental health charity 42nd street, and also worked as a part of the Midlands Young Advisors. They passionately advocate for better mental healthcare for children and young people from an LGBTQ+ perspective.

Stuart Dodzo has been advocating for young people's involvement in service co-design since a long-term health condition diagnosis at 17, which provided first-hand experience of accessing physical and mental health services as a young person from a minoritised background. His public involvement experience includes: co-production coordinator at Healthy Teen Minds, NIHR MindTech Advisory Group member, panel member of CQC Closed Cultures Expert Advisory Group, University College London COVID19 trials Patient and Public Involvement (PPI) group and Public Advisory Group for the Evidence Synthesis Centre (University of Sheffield and National Institute of Health Research).

Demi is an expert by experience of over 10 years. She now has an understanding of herself since gaining an autism diagnosis and has a successful career as a technologist. Since beginning her career, Demi has received an apprentice of the year award and is embarking on a leadership programme aimed at supporting women in leadership roles. Demi maintains a connection with mental health by working behind the scenes supporting a parent-carer support group founded by her mum.

Harry Dixon has worked in the mental healthcare sector since 2016 whilst studying for his undergraduate degree in Digital Film and Television Production. During his studies, he passionately worked to become a peer support worker at his local child and adolescent mental health service, and became a member of the Midlands Young Advisors. He is currently training as an Education Mental Health Practitioner.

Sarah Gray is a social worker, play therapist, EMDR therapist, specialist eating disorder therapist, systemic family practitioner and clinical supervisor with over 40 years of experience in the field of Child Mental Health. Sarah is the Clinical Lead for South Derbyshire CAMHS and has a private practice as a Play Therapist. Sarah is passionate about participation and co-production having been promoting the voice of the child since working with a group of care leavers in the late 1980s.

Sarah currently manages the CAMHS Participation Team, which consists of young people and parents employed by the service.

Oli Hawley is a peer consultant at ImROC who specialises in children and young people's peer support and participation, and in inclusive and equitable approaches to mental health work and education. He was a member of the Midlands Young Advisors for five years, during which time he rose to co-lead the team. Beyond this, Oli offers consultancy and project management to other mental health and recovery projects, across to NHS and partner organisations across the Midlands. He hopes to further apply his interest in equitable support through a masters in inclusive education.

Sarah Hutchins has worked in Derbyshire in the lived experience field within Child and Adolescent Mental Health Services (CAMHS). She has used her personal experience of using this service to support young people through a CAMHS participation group and to shape and develop new services for young people. A project which the CAMHS participation group is particularly proud of is co-producing an event to raise awareness for World Mental Health Day in 2022. She has achieved a first-class BSc in Psychology from The Open University and aims to continue her studies to become an Occupational Therapist within Children's Services.

Duncan Law is visiting professor at University College London's Department of Clinical, Educational and Health Psychology. A Consultant Clinical Psychologist with over 30 years of experience working across child and adult mental health settings. He is Director of MindMonkey Associates, currently working on research and transformation programmes in the UK, Canada, and Scandinavia. He teaches at the Anna Freud Centre where he was clinical lead for children and young people's IAPT for London and the Southeast. He is a practicing clinician with an interest in collaborative practice and is the developer of the goals-based outcome (GBO) tool.

Rachel McGuire is a parent/carer, with over a decade of expert experience, who is passionate about improving children and young people's mental health and supporting families. She advocates the benefits of, and actively engages in, working with all parties connected to family life, from communities and services to policy, in order to evaluate needs and provide the best support available. She currently works as a researcher on studies led by the Anna Freud National Centre for Children and Families and the Norfolk and Suffolk Foundation Trust. She worked with the co-production team during the development of Lumi Nova – a NICE approved therapeutic mobile game for children – and now builds case studies liaising with families who use it.

Wendy Minhinnett is a parent with lived experience who has been involved in a variety of initiatives locally and nationally to promote the role parents can play in improving children and young people's mental health (CYPMH). Wendy is a co-founder of Rollercoaster Parent Support Project, is the Parent Lead for the Charlie Waller Trust and coordinates the PLACE CYPMH National Network of parent-carer support projects. Wendy believes in a parent-led, professionally supported model of practice and hopes for a future where every family has access to the support and information they need to support their child's mental health.

Carol-Anne Murphy is a Nurse Consultant in Children and Young People's Mental Health Services. She has worked across inpatient, community, and youth offending teams as well as focusing on transitions to adult services. Having worked in the sector for over 35 years, she also holds a Masters qualification in leadership and management and a PGCE in higher education as well as currently being Chair of the Quality Network for Community CAMHS (QNCC) Advisory Committee.

Lucy North works as a People Participation Lead at Norfolk and Suffolk NHS Foundation Trust (NSFT). Lucy knows first-hand the importance of having the voices of children, young people, parents and carers at the heart of everything in the field. Lucy has previously been a Peer Support Worker and has a vision to actively involve as many people with lived experience in participation as possible.

Kathryn Pugh MBE has spent over 20 years working to improve children and young people's mental health services. Her roles include commissioning, service development, and as part of VCSE organisations. As Head of Policy at YoungMinds she instigated changes to the Mental Health Act regarding age-appropriate environments, which she then implemented for the UK government. At NHS England she led many aspects of the community CYPMH Transformation Programme including CYP IAPT, Future in Mind, Transforming Children and Young People's Mental Health – Green Paper and the NHS Long Term Plan. She has her own lived experience, both as an individual and parent. In 2015, she was awarded an MBE for services to children and young people's mental health.

Zaynab "ZeZe" Sohawon is an multi-award-winning children and young people's mental health advocate and lived experience practitioner. She holds various lived-experience roles, including as a mental health and autism lived experience advisor, and a psychosis lived experience consultant. She is currently pursuing a degree in human neuroscience with a view to pursuing a career in psychiatry.

Cathy Street is an Honorary Associate Professor at Warwick Medical School. She was previously the Patient and Public Involvement (PPI) Lead for The MILESTONE Project, a pan-European research study looking at young people's mental health service transitions, where Warwick Medical School was one of the research sites. Over the last 20 years, both across the UK and internationally, Cathy has worked to promote co-production with young people with lived experience in mental health research, evaluation, and service improvement activities.

The Midlands Young Advisors are a group of young people who provide consultancy and advocacy services relating to children and young people's participation in mental health services. They were formed in 2017 as part of the Children and Young People's Improving Access to Psychological Therapies programme. The team consists of up to 14 children and young people aged between 16 and 25, based in the Midlands region, with experiences of mental health challenges, service access, and/or a passion for improving children and young people's mental health services.

Trafford Youth Cabinet is a local youth council which forms part of the British Youth Council. They work with young people who live, work, or go to school in Trafford on a range of social issues. A key area of their focus is improving mental health support for young people, having ran multiple campaigns and conferences on the topic in recent years. Their members have gone on to successfully take up roles on national mental health projects.

Anna Wilson is an expert-by-experience in the children and young people's mental health field. She has passionately advocated for better participation in children and young people's mental health services since 2014. Her experiences have led to her pursuing a career in medicine where she continues to work to make services the best they can be.

Foreword

Most forewords are written by one person. But the editors asked the four of us to write this together as between us we represent everyone who needs to read this book and take the advice of the authors of each chapter. We reflect direct experiences as young people, parents, professionals, service leaders, commissioners, and as policy makers. Between us we have delivered, influenced, and seen change happen, but know that more is needed to finally establish participation and co-production as essential to delivery of reflective, excellent services that meet the needs of those they serve.

We have written our own reflections separately but iteratively, with each other's drafts sparking off conversations, shaping our final joint approach.

Stuart Dodzo (He/Him), Young Person with Lived Experience, Co-production Coordinator

As a young person with lived experience, committed to ensuring young people are involved in service co-design to help shape services for young people and people with long-term health conditions, I am pleased to see tools, such as this book, becoming more accessible, and young people, present and in the future, who are interested in getting involved in co-production exercises within mental health services have evidence when asking for adjustments. We are not being unreasonable when asking for adjustments or calling out bad practice!

My experience of co-production is influenced by my personal experience and involvement in national advisory groups for a range of organisations including the Care Quality Commission (CQC), National Institute of Health Research (NIHR) and the Mental Health Foundation.

Chapter 3 explores the difference between tokenism and meaningful engagement and for people who have been affected by life-changing experiences tokenism can add insult to injury, lead to lack of trust in services, makes the work less legitmate, and hinders spaces that should harness authenticity through trust and openness. Legitimacy of the work (involvement and participation) is something I struggled with in the early stages of my young people's involvement journey. I had healthcare work experience and some certificates to cover my academic credentials. However, from my lived experience, I thought I had nothing. Questions I still have whilst typing this: How do lived experience contributors measure the legitimacy of their work? What are researchers and health professionals' opinions on the legitimacy of lived-experience work? It is good to see research around this work and interest from professionals. In Chapter 4 we read about the benefits of participation for patients. It is important to capture first-hand accounts, as feedback, of participation from the individuals involved. Participation can be difficult, and I believe all those involved in it understand this, but it should be a positive experience for all involved (and the services impacted).

In my commitment to young people's involvement, 'sustainability' is a very important aspect/factor to consider in this and this can only be achieved through systemic culture change. Chapter 14 consolidates the argument that the only way to achieve the change towards meaningful participation, which is called for is to systematically change the culture of CYPMHs.

Young people should have a voice in service development. This book guides services and young people on how they should be involved at different levels through co-production.

Rachel McGuire (She/Her), Parent, and Expert by Lived Experience

Parents, carers, and young people who have accessed support from mental health services feel they have a depth of knowledge and understanding which is quite different from that of professionals. As a parent of a child I have supported over the last decade, with her mental health challenges, I call myself an expert by lived experience. This book recognises that through experience, parents and carers have learned how to advocate for their children and how to help professionals fully understand the difficulties.

Chapter 13 discusses the idea that those who have walked similar paths can teach and learn collaboratively. Through peer support and relationships, which are based on growing together, we are empowered to share our insights. With training, those who might feel they have become estranged through anxiety or depression and a lack of self-confidence has crept in, are equipped, and enabled to find a new purpose and self-identity.

Chapters 6 and 7 recognise that being involved in the care of a young person is about how to surround them with meaningful support that comes from joint decisions made by themselves, their parents or carers and the professionals in charge of their care. What a relief when the result is a care plan that works for the young person at home, school and within their social world! Chapter 9 goes beyond a parent or carer's personal experience to highlight opportunities in improving services for others. Participation in a formal capacity within research, for me as parent advisor and co-producer, means equal partnership. This book demonstrates how this can be done, not only through consultation, but recognised contributions being made every step of the way.

This book, which has been produced by two young people who have lived some of their best experiences through participation alongside professionals, proves we are moving in a direction where participation matters to many; that feels exciting. When a parent/carer is championed to participate in their child's care in a way that gets right to the heart of meeting their child's needs, something magical happens. Each chapter is an important read for those of us supporting a young person living with mental health challenges and for all our allies playing a major role in supporting us along the way.

Duncan Law (He/Him), Consult Clinical Psychologist and Visiting Professor at University College London's Department of Clinical, Education and Health Psychology

As a clinician and academic, my primary concern is how to provide the best possible clinical practices within the most appropriately organised mental health services. How to ensure we make best use of the limited resources that are available to us in the children and young people's mental health (CYPMH) system. The question is always: 'how do we best do this?' Over the past decade, collaboration, participation, and co-production, with the young people, their parents and carers, and the communities in which they live, have increasingly become seen as a vital and necessary part of the answer.

This book provides an enormous contribution to answering that question, 'what does good participation look like in practice?' Chapter 6 looks at the central clinical issue of involving young people in their own care. The benefits of which are well known but the practice of which is less well embedded in therapy services. Chapter 4 looks of the wider benefits of participation on the mental health of those who participate. Which helpfully challenges the notion that mental health professionals are the best and only route to recovery. Chapter 9 gives an overview of how best to involve young people in the complex and bureaucratic world of research. Chapters 11 and 10, tackle the complexities of hearing those seldom-heard voices of young people in diverse communities and the voice of younger children. These chapters remind us that in order to have services that are equitable, accessible, and acceptable to all, participation must draw on the widest range of views and experiences. Chapter 14 tackles the need for culture change, to really value participation and co-production.

Culture change is always complex; however, culture is held by people and culture change starts with changing ourselves. It reminds us to break from the traditionally assigned roles of 'professional' and 'patient', with all the implicit imbalance of power that come with them, and see ourselves as people collaborating with other people, sharing expertise to get to a better place.

Of course, the most compelling chapters are the ones where we hear the authentic voice of those with lived experience of children and young people's mental health system, be it as children and young people themselves, or their parents and carers. If professionals are genuinely interested in providing best clinical practice, then these are the voices we must listen to.

Kathryn Pugh (She/Her), Former Deputy Head of Mental Health NHS England – Children and Young People Community Transformation

This is the book I wish I had when I first started commissioning children and young people's mental health services – and how useful would it have been in the years since when I have worked in the voluntary sector, then for the NHS on service development and change at a national and regional level. For the last 20 years, although I have done everything I could to ensure children, young people and their families were fully involved in every aspect of their own experience of accessing a service, from what happens 'in the room' through to service design, realising authentic participation has been an uphill struggle. So, have things changed? Or are we just getting better at lip service? Despite the work of the National CAMHS Support Service, CYP IAPT, and Future in Mind programmes, authentic participation is in so many parts of the country still fragile and even the best systems can lose it either through complacency, neglect, or ignorance. The promise of 'No decision about me, without me'[1] was coined in the last period of austerity, but unless we meet real need in a way that works for those who want to use them, we cannot move forwards.

This is an optimistic book, embracing practical as well as theoretical and academic aspects (Chapter 2 and 3). So if you are trying to involve younger age children (Chapter 10), if you want to improve your service (Chapter 5 and 8), really begin to tackle getting representative voices from your community – including parents (Chapter 3 and 11), involve young people in research (Chapter 9) or writing a business case you will find information here.

But, to my professional, commissioning and policy colleagues I want to add a word of caution. Reliving their past – and their present – so that we might learn lessons from their positive and negative journeys can be painful and distressing, so please respect, support, and appreciate the generosity of our experts and their hard-won experience.

Stuart, Rachel, Duncan, and Kathryn

We want to congratulate you for buying and reading this book – it will provide you with inspiration, practical tips, and the knowledge that there is a community of good people out there who want the best for our children, young people, their families, and the professionals that aim every day to help. But in order for participation and co-production – and these services – to thrive, every one of us needs to continue to ask difficult questions, some of us cede power, others step forward and demand an equal share of that power. We recommend that for whatever reason you bought this book that you try to read each chapter and commit to doing everything you can to support its aims.

Stuart Dodzo (He/Him), young person with lived experience, co-production coordinator
Rachel McGuire (She/Her), parent and expert by lived experience
Duncan Law (He/Him), Consult Clinical Psychologist and Visiting Professor at University College London's Department of Clinical, Education and Health Psychology
Kathryn Pugh (She/Her), former Deputy Head of Mental Health NHS England – Children and Young People Community Transformation

Note

1 Liberating the NHS: No decision about me, without me (publishing.service. gov.uk).

Acknowledgements

We cannot express enough how thankful we are to every single person who has contributed to this book. Thank you for your knowledge, wisdom, time, and commitment to the vision. Particularly to those who have so vulnerably shared their own lived experiences, we know how much courage and strength it can take.

Thank you to the people in our lives who have supported us through our own hard times, we appreciate you so much.

Chapter 1

Introduction

Hannah Sharp (She/Her) and
Leanne Walker (She/They)

A Introduction to the Editors

Leanne Walker (She/They) PGCert, BA (Hons)

Participation changed my life. I might even go as far as saying it saved my life.

I first accessed young people's mental health services at age 15 experiencing a range of difficulties including depression, anxiety, and self-harm. I did not leave the service until I was 19 years old and in that time I had a range of interventions to treat what I was experiencing. I was often described as 'complex' and one problem turned into another.

My mental health records talk about the mental health worker I saw, the youth group I went to, and the therapy I received, but there is little to no mention of participation. There is no documentation of the positive impact participation had on my life, nor no means to capture the massive ongoing ripples of participation that I am still feeling to this day, 10 years after first joining the participation group. For me, I needed the years of work with my mental health worker to get to a place where I could trust others, to be able to communicate what I was experiencing, and talk openly. This enabled me to then be able to do therapy and I needed the therapy to work through my social anxiety to be able to then attend the services participation group.

It was the combination and order of these things that enabled me to be in a place to engage in participation that led for such a massive shift for me.

Participation enabled me to take all the negative, really difficult things I had experienced and turn them into something positive. It gave me a voice, showed me what I had to say had value and that I mattered. It showed me the world would miss me if I was not in it and that I had a place here on this earth. It gave me purpose.

My mental health worker came with me to my first participation group to support me. I did not have any idea then, what a life changing moment

DOI: 10.4324/9781003288800-1

that was to be for me and I remain grateful to them in so many ways to this day.

In that group I developed a lot of skills. I was able to test out and put into practise what I was learning in therapy in a safe environment. I could not get on a bus before, but in this space I learnt how to speak in front of audiences. I developed social skills and my confidence grew and, critically for me, I made friends. When I speak about the impact participation had on me, I talk about the lifelong impact of making friends who you feel understand you, are there for you, and are people you can call upon during the worst and best times. There are five of us who all connected through participation and, to the present day, we remain close. This has been, and continues to be, an ongoing ripple of participation within my life. I also stayed involved in participation after I was discharged from the service, making leaving feel easier and safer.

In 2013, as a participation group member, I spoke at a conference for the first time about my lived experiences of mental health difficulties. Within the audience was an organisation called GIFT (Great Involvement Future Thinking) who employed young people on a sessional basis to do participation work nationally. I joined the team shortly after and from then I have held various advisory and lived experience roles within the mental health field and have engaged with work locally, nationally, and internationally. For five years I even worked in the same young people's mental health service I used myself, running the participation groups I used to go to. Combined, this has given me a full-circle perspective and participation continues to play such an important role in my life. Currently I am working in a lived experience role at Derbyshire Healthcare NHS Foundation Trust.

Hannah Sharp (She/Her), BA(Hons)

My journey with participation started when I was 14 (I'm now 23 at the time of writing) before I'd even accessed services myself. I saw friends struggle and it broke my heart knowing there were systemic issues which I could see solutions to. I then began to struggle with my own mental health, and I believe participation played a critical role in helping keep me out of hospital.

Participation gave me purpose and it gave me something to look forward to. It taught me I was valued and my life had value – I was able to make something better.

Through my involvement in local initiatives and then national and international policy, I grew as a person. When I look back at the recording of my first conference presentation, I am timid, lack autonomy, look around for reassurance, and, in general, seem low. Now, I am able to stand in front of a room of 300+ people and confidently tell my story.

During this time, I became interested in making participation itself better. I saw its value, but I saw its problems. Eventually my knowledge on participation grew to a point where I was speaking not just about my own experience, but about participation in general and its flaws. One thing led to another and eventually I found myself, a 15-year-old still struggling with raging depression, stood in front of a conference at the European Parliament telling people about participation and its best practice. Since then, I have been involved in a number of high-profile events and projects. I am now studying for a PhD in mental health so I can continue to make a difference for those with mental health difficulties.

Over the years, as I've progressed down my recovery journey, I can now see how important participation was in that recovery. As I have mentioned, the purpose and motivation it gave me provided me with hope and a desire to be better. I would not be who I am today without participation. I wholeheartedly believe that.

But there is still so much progress to be made and that's why this book is important. I know what participation did for me, and I know what it can do for other people. We need to keep pushing to improve participation and therefore amplify its impact. It can play a critical part in someone's therapeutic journey, just like it did with mine, as well as making services more effective for everyone.

Introduction to the Text

This text acts as a comprehensive exploration of and guide to participation in the children and young people's mental health (CYPMH) field. It is also certainly the case that many of its lessons can be applied to participation in adult and older adult services too, though throughout the text we place an emphasis on the unique challenges of participation with children and young people (CYP), parents, and carers. It explores topics from how we conceptualise participation to more practical advice and guidance surrounding how we actually 'do' participation. We would like to particularly point colleagues towards the chapters written by people with lived experience. Some of the most powerful lessons come from hearing directly from the experience of those who, like us, have been through it themselves. If there are any chapters you read in this text, it should be those.

We hope you enjoy reading, and take lessons away with you to embed in your services, organisations, areas, groups, practice, and work. We hope to spark thinking, conversations, and actions. Participation is not easy, otherwise we'd have it sorted already and there would be no need for this text. By following this text's guidance however, we hope you can make strong and positive steps towards making it obsolete. Our goal is for this text to no longer be necessary, because participation is fully embedded in everyone's practice across the field.

Why 'CYPMH'?

We chose CYPMH instead of Child and Adolescent Mental Health Services (CAMHS), firstly because we wanted to be inclusive of all of the CYP mental health field, be it services, organisations or groups (etc). We want to acknowledge the important role of the voluntary sector and private providers in ensuring their service users also benefit from participation. Secondly and critically, in our experience and the experiences of colleagues we have spoken with, the 'adolescent' in CAMHS has become outdated with many CYP finding it patronising. 'CYPMH' emerged instead and is now commonly being used to refer to CYP mental health or CYPMHS to refer to Children and Young People's Mental Health Services.

A Note on Participation Versus Co-Production

Throughout this text, the term 'participation' is primarily used. We wish here to comment on the concept of co-production. Co-production should be the goal of quality participation – whereby patients, parents, and carers are involved in the participation process from before conception right through to review. Therefore, when we talk about 'participation' throughout this text we are mindful that co-production is often seen as the 'gold standard' when it comes to participation. We have chosen to use the term 'participation' partly because of the Children and Young People's Improving Access to Psychological Therapies (CYP IAPT) transformation, which shone a spotlight onto what was termed 'participation' as core to CYPMHS. We are also realistic that where services and the field are at means that co-production is not viable for every opportunity. We do not wish to exclude the important work that goes on where perhaps participants have not come up with the idea themselves. For example, participation in interviews or annual service evaluations. So, co-production, or the emerging phrase 'co-creation' is the goal and when we refer to participation in an aspirational sense, this is what we are referring to.

The Statutory Requirement to 'Involve'

This book is not just about participation as something which is a 'nice to have' or just something with benefits for service users, parent/carers, staff, and services themselves. There exists a statutory duty to, as NHS England (2022) and the new Health and Care Act (2022) term it, 'involve'. This latest act creates a particularly exciting time for participation.

The Act extends the remit of those who must be involved as set out in the National Health Service Act (2006) to include parents and carers. This is a significant step forward in recognising the important role that parent/carers play in the care of those they care for. In our experience, this role is particularly important in CYP mental healthcare whereby parent/carers can even be involved in part of the therapeutic interventions, such as family therapy, but also recognising often it is parents/carer who know their child best.

The 2022 Act also strengthens the duty to involve patients in decisions about their own health via prevention, involvement in treatment, and patient choice. In addition, it stipulates that new Integrated Care Boards (ICBs) must involve patients and parent/carers in commissioning – entrenching historic requirements to involve patients and the public in commissioning in this new system.

It also highlights the importance of innovation and research. We argue throughout this text that participation is key in meeting this statutory duty, as well as providing practical advice and guidance on how to meet these requirements.

Perhaps most importantly, it requires NHS England to include public involvement and consultation in the yearly evaluations of the performance of Integrated Care Boards (ICBs). This, therefore, is not just part of the act which can be 'swept under the carpet'.

The problem with this guidance however, is its use of the term 'involve' without any real definition of what 'involve' constitutes. This is where a text like this becomes important.

A Brief History of Participation Policy in Children and Young People's Mental Health Services (CYPMHS)

The journey for participation in CYPMHS to get to where it is today has been turbulent.

When discussing the policy change leading up to this conception of participation in CYPMHS, there are three key policy journeys to discuss. The first is the journey of participation in the UK National Health Service (NHS) more broadly, the second is changing attitudes in mental healthcare towards a focus on community care and patient autonomy, and the third is the increasing emphasis on the voice of the child.

The concept of patient participation began to emerge onto the policy agenda in the 1970s with a shift towards a neoliberalist political ideology. The marketisation of public services gave rise to participation framed within consumerism as a tool for increasing service efficiency. Prior to this there was an undercurrent of interest in participation, but there were no significant policies that supported it (Beresford, 2020). In addition to a change in the political philosophy of the State, the public began to demonstrate an increasing dissatisfaction with service provision (Croft and Beresford, 1992; Beresford, 2020). New social movements that challenged the traditional power of public institutions over service provision began to gain traction (Croft and Beresford, 1992). These movements were determined to democratise the health system such that their needs were met. They were not concerned with the broader system and politics of health, they wanted their right to have support acknowledged and to be an equal partner to clinicians (Beresford, 2020; Bowl, 1996).

The 1980s and 1990s began to see some small successes for the public and those pushing for greater participation. Notably, the 1991 Patient's Charter was committed to an NHS that was more responsive to the needs of its patients, a commitment echoed in the 2009 NHS Constitution, which remains in place today with slight updates (Stocking, 1991; Department of Health, 2021). The rhetoric surrounding patient participation had developed from a focus on public consultation into one surrounding user-centred, individualised care (Bowl, 1996). There was however, little effort to ensure that participation was inclusive and representative (Croft and Beresford, 1992) and the public remained a tokenistic tool used to 'legitimate, rather than challenge, existing provision' (Rhodes and Nocon, 1998, p.73).

The 2000s–2010s saw the publication of two key reports investigating unsafe practices within the NHS, which highlighted the role participation ought to play in helping to resolve them. The Bristol Royal Infirmary Inquiry (2001) into the avoidable deaths of over 30 children being treated on the cardiac unit at The Bristol Royal Infirmary between 1991 and 1995 highlighted the need for a change in power structures and accountability in the NHS. A large group of the 198 recommendations made by the report surrounded patient participation (Chambers, Drinkwater and Boath, 2003). Twelve years later, the publication of a report investigating significant failures by the Mid Staffordshire NHS Foundation Trust which resulted in an estimated 400 to 1,200 deaths highlighted similar concerns. It argued that there were systemic failures in how participation was facilitated and made several recommendations for improving the patient's voice. One such recommendation was that 'there must be real involvement of patients and the public in all that is done' (Francis, 2013, p.74). The recommendations made in both reports are concerningly similar, indicating that no real change was made in relation to participation as a result of the Bristol Enquiry. Therefore, it can be concluded that even significant and widely publicised events were not enough to drive strong changes in patient participation policy.

This is a very brief and thus limited overview of the development of participation policy prior to 2011. While there are other documents and events, which could add to the discussion, its purpose is to show simply that despite a continued policy commitment to improving participation, progress was slow, incremental, and limited.

The second key policy journey is that of changing attitudes in mental healthcare towards a focus on community care and patient autonomy. Like the development of participation, deinstitutionalisation was partially driven by the voice of service users who called for greater humanity towards mental health patients (The King's Fund, 2015a). Furthermore, developments in the treatment of mental illness using medication meant that it was easier and, in fact, more conducive to recovery to treat patients in the community (The King's Fund, 2015a). The 1962 Hospital Plan facilitated the further development of community mental health services (CMHS) and reconfigured inpatient services to be focused on shorter, and more targeted admissions (Turner et al., 2015). However, due to CMHS being poorly developed, the first closure of an asylum directly resulting from the plan was not until 1986, some 24 years later (The King's Fund, 2015a).

The ability for mental health patients detained by law to appeal their detention via a tribunal was introduced as part of the 1983 reformation of The Mental Health Act and was founded upon a recognition that detention was a serious loss of liberty, which the patient had a right to challenge (Wood, 1993). These changes, amongst others within the reform, helped to make patients a stronger partner in their care.

While the closure of asylums took over 24 years to begin to take place, the early 2000s saw a rapid period of change within CMHS. Public pressure to improve these services resulting from a number of high-profile incidents helped to introduce a 47% increase (in real terms) in funding for CMHSs between 1999/2000 and 2005/06 (The King's Fund, 2015b). A high number of new services were to be set-up using this funding, though full implementation was never reached. Furthermore, data collected showed underperformance of services and overly optimistic cuts in inpatient bed capacity put excessive pressure on inpatient services, causing acuity in the community to rise and increasing pressure on CMHS (The King's Fund, 2015b).

Deinstitutionalisation exemplifies the changing attitude that mental health patients are capable of autonomy. Patients who once would have been committed to a lifetime locked inside the asylum where decisions were made about them, became respected as capable of making rational decisions, and thus became candidates to meaningfully engage in participation. Therefore, deinstitutionalisation is a critical part of the journey of participation in mental health services. It also shows that rapid and comprehensive reform is possible when the right circumstances are present.

In tandem with these changes, there was a similar shift occurring towards the recognition of CYP as citizens with a right and ability to make choices about what happens to them. The new sociology of childhood emerging in the 1980s and 1990s (Quennerstedt and Quennerstedt, 2014) and the publication of the United Nations Convention on the Rights of the Child (UNCRC) in 1989 (UN General Assembly, 1989) stimulated a political and social shift toward recognising children as individual agents (Solberg, 2015).

Article 12 of the UNCRC states that:

> States Parties shall assure to the child who is capable of forming his or her own views the right to express those views freely in all matters affecting the child, the views of the child being given due weight in accordance with the age and maturity of the child.

This encompasses the right for children to have a say in decisions made about their healthcare. This was emphasised in UK policy as part of the 'National Service Framework for Children, Young People and Maternity Services', which stressed that CYP, even those who are 'very young', ought to be included in service development (Department of Health, 2004). The introduction of the use of the 'Gillick Competence' in 1986 to assess a child's capacity to consent has supported those under the age of 16 to make decisions about their own healthcare and is now used as standard throughout CYPMHS (Care Quality Commission, 2019). However, stigma still existed and parents remained the default decision-makers in their child's care (Anderson and Sharp, 2020).

To summarise, by 2011 there had been slow progress towards an emphasis in policy on patient participation. Mental health patients were being viewed as more capable of decision making and there was notable recognition of the role that children ought to play in decision making. These three policy areas converge into what we understand as CYPMHS policy.

The rest of this text will largely focus on CYPMHS policy post-2011. So, we will leave this discussion here and move on to the present.

References

Anderson, Y. and Sharp, H. (2020). Children's Participation: Making it happen. In: Kick-off participatie in de geestelijke gezondheidszorg: 1ste WEBINAR 7 december 2020. 2020. [Online] Available at: https://www.health.belgium.be/nl/agenda/participatie-van-kinderen-en-jongeren-en-hun-context-de-geestelijke-gezondheidszorg.

Beresford, P. (2020). PPI or User Involvement: Taking stock from a service user perspective in the twenty first century. *Research Involvement and Engagement*, 6 (1), BioMed Central Ltd. [Online] Available at: doi:10.1186/s40900-020-00211-8.

Bowl, R. (1996). Legislating for user involvement in the United Kingdom: Mental health services and the NHS and Community Care Act 1990. *International Journal of Social Psychiatry*, 42 (3), pp.165–180. [Online] Available at: doi:10.1177/002076409604200301.

Care Quality Commission (2019). *Brief Guide: Capacity and Competence to Consent in Under 18s.* [Online]. CQC. Last updated: July 2020. Available at: https://www.cqc.org.uk/sites/default/files/Brief_guide_Capacity_and_consent_in_under_18s%20v3.pdf [Accessed 26 January 2023].

Chambers, R., Drinkwater, C. and Boath, E. (2003). *Involving Patients and the Public - How to do it better.* Oxon: Radcliffe Medical Press.

Croft, S. and Beresford, P. (1992). The politics of participation. *Critical Social Policy*, 12 (35), pp.20–44. [Online] Available at: doi:10.1177/026101839201203502 [Accessed 16 October 2020].

Department of Health (2004). National service framework for children, young people and maternity services. [Online] Available at: http://www.dh.gov.uk/Pol icyAndGuidance/HealthAndSocialCareTopics/ChildrenServices/fs/en [Accessed 16 May 2021].

Department of Health (2021). The NHS Constitution for England. [Online] Available at: https://www.gov.uk/government/publications/the-nhs-constitution-for-england/ the-nhs-constitution-for-england [Accessed 26 February 2021].

Francis, R. (2013). Report of the Mid Staffordshire NHS Foundation Trust Public Inquiry. Crown copyright. [Online] Available at: doi:10.1002/yd.20044 [Accessed 24 May 2021].

Health and Care Act (2022).

NHS England (2022). *Working in partnership with people and communities: Statutory guidance.* [Online]. NHS England. Last Updated: 10 October 2022. Available at: https://www.england.nhs.uk/long-read/working-in-partnership -with-people-and-communities-statutory-gu [Accessed 26 January 2023].

Quennerstedt, A. and Quennerstedt, M. (2014). Researching children's rights in education: sociology of childhood encountering educational theory. *British Journal of Sociology of Education*, 35 (1), pp.115–132. [Online] Available at: doi:10.1080/01425692.2013.783962 [Accessed 11 May 2021].

Rhodes, P. and Nocon, A. (1998). User involvement and the NHS reforms. *Health Expectations*, 1 (2), pp.73–81. [Online] Available at: doi:10.1046/j.1369-6513.1998.00021.x.

Solberg, A. (2015). Negotiating Childhood. Changing constructions of age for Norwegian Children. In: James, A. and Prout, A. (Eds). *Constructing and reconstructing childhood: Contemporary issues in the sociological study of childhood.* Routledge, pp.111–127.

Stocking, B. (1991). Patient's charter. *British Medical Journal*, 303 (6811), British Medical Journal Publishing Group, pp.1148–1149. [Online] Available at: doi:10.1136/bmj.303.6811.1148 [Accessed 10 May 2021].

The Bristol Royal Infirmary Inquiry (2001). *The Report of the Public Inquiry into children's heart surgery at the Bristol Royal Infirmary 1984–1995 - Learning from Bristol.* The Stationary Office.

The King's Fund (2015a). Case study 1: Deinstitutionalisation in UK mental health services. [Online] Available at: https://www.kingsfund.org.uk/publica tions/making-change-possible/mental-health-services [Accessed 10 May 2021].

The King's Fund (2015b). Case study 2: The National Service Framework for Mental Health in England. [Online] Available at: https://www.kingsfund.org. uk/publications/making-change-possible/national-service-framework-mental-he alth-england [Accessed 10 May 2021].

Turner, J. *et al.* (2015). The history of mental health services in modern England: Practitioner memories and the direction of future research. *Medical History*, 59 (4), Cambridge University Press, pp.599–624. [Online] Available at: doi:10.1017/ mdh.2015.48 [Accessed 11 May 2021].

UN General Assembly (1989). *The United Nations Convention on the Rights of the Child*. United Nations.

Wood, J. (1993). Reform of the Mental Health Act 1983. An effective tribunal system. *British Journal of Psychiatry*, 162 (JAN.), Cambridge University Press, pp.14–22. [Online] Available at: doi:10.1192/bjp.162.1.14 [Accessed 11 May 2021].

Chapter 2

What is Participation? A Theoretical Framework for Children and Young People's Participation

Yvonne Anderson

Introduction

How can we synthesise and articulate the guiding principles and core ideas of children and young people's participation? Many of the contributors to this book describe in detail the various practices of participation, its benefits, and how to evaluate them. In this chapter I propose a framework as the basis for future theory on children's and young people's participation, creating the rationale by reviewing related literature and ideas, and relating them to lived experience.

Participation has many definitions and connotations. Young people entering university are described as 'participating in education', belonging to a local hockey team is seen as 'participating in sport', attending an art gallery, musical concert, or museum might be understood as 'participating in culture' (Leguina & Miles 2017). These may be termed 'lifestyle participation'. We, however, are concerned here with the more specific meaning of participation, which can be characterised as involvement that influences decision-making and challenges orthodox power structures. Our focus is the participation of children and young people in all areas that affect them in our largely adult-led world.

Against the backdrop of universal children's rights, much of the published work on children's participation has been set in an international context. The internationally focused papers referenced here provide rich context as well as widely applicable themes. This chapter is focused on the UK and on countries and regions that share similarities to the UK. The specific emphasis here is on participation by children and young people in the services they use. Despite that emphasis I believe that readers from a range of other participation settings will find much that relates to them, and while I make no claims for international applicability, I hope the framework will have relevance and be generalisable across wider domains.

(The words 'child' and 'children' are used throughout this chapter to include infants, children, and adolescents/young people.)

DOI: 10.4324/9781003288800-2

The Importance of Theory and its Relationship to Practice

A simple understanding of theory and practice is that theory is thinking about something, and practice is doing something. Put that way they seem to be very different propositions. But there would be little point in unthinking practice; doing without thinking can be dangerous. Likewise, theory about humans is empty and meaningless unless it is applied to practice. In this sense, theory and practice are co-dependent and have equal value.

Theory gives shape to sets of ideas and principles that we hold, based on our observations of the world. In simple theories the observations may be casual and unstructured, whereas more complex theories are based upon systematic and sometimes scientific methods of observation, making them more elaborate and detailed.

The plethora of models and typologies in children's participation has created plenty of guidance for practice. This, however, has been at the expense of any underpinning theory and as a consequence has helped to create an understanding of children's participation that is more procedural than strategic, and more practical than intellectual. In other words: children's participation is generally defined by how it is done and the field has progressed by the use of evolving models of practice. This is problematic because the absence of theory denotes an absence of meaning and children's participation must have meaning if it is to have value and be seen to have value. Additionally, theory is a starting point for research and research provides evidence of outcomes. While the process of participating may be a valuable experience in itself, it is to the outcomes, the benefits, and tangible results that we now need to look.

Constructs of Children and Children's Participation

Children and young people have specific needs and wishes that will often be different from those of adults. That said, the needs and wishes of all people are in a constant state of change, throughout all phases or stages of a lifetime. Interests and concerns at age 10 will be very different once we reach 20, but the difference may be equally pronounced between the ages of 30 and 40, or 50 and 60. A theory for the participation of children and young people must take account of pre-existing theories of childhood and human development, not just those concerned with psychosocial development (See: Cherry 2022 on Piaget and Cherry 2021 on Erikson) but also those that differentiate infant, child, and adolescent neuro-development from that of adults (Casey et al. 2008, Tierney & Nelson 2009).

Theories of infant, child, and adolescent development are helpful in the development of a theory of participation in as much as they underline differences in need and spheres of interest. The caveat to that is opposition to the use of such theories to construct concepts of children's 'capacity', since in the context of participation we need only be concerned with their capability. Children of all ages and abilities are capable of knowing what they need and like. This is illustrated amply by this description of a young child by Alderson et al. (2006: 30):

> At 3 years, Maisie warned her mother when she was feeling hypo (shaky from low blood sugar). At 4 years, Ruby could be trusted not to eat chocolates when her friend did and no adults were nearby, and by 5 she could test her blood sugar level and decide how much cake she could eat at a birthday party.

Children and young people are often not heard or taken seriously and this is well illustrated in a brief history. For centuries in the UK and elsewhere, children were seen as the responsibility of their parents and families with no intervention from church or state. Children had no protections beyond what their families and immediate communities would provide. In largely agrarian communities children worked more or less the same hours as adults. Industrialisation initiated massive social change that included a growing concern for the welfare of children, reflected in child labour reforms and some children's rights such as to basic education. The resultant child welfare charities focused on 'saving' disadvantaged children, with the result that children were taken from their families including many who were shipped thousands of miles to work in servitude in other countries. Home Children was the child migration scheme in which more than 100,000 children were sent from the United Kingdom to Australia, Canada, New Zealand, and South Africa. While the programme was mostly discontinued in the 1930s, it did not end entirely until the 1970s. The voice of the child in all of this was not even considered.

The 20th century saw the responsibility for children's welfare shift towards greater state involvement, but only in the second half of that century did the idea start to take hold of children having agency and holding citizens' rights. In 1924, the League of Nations adopted the Geneva Declaration on the Rights of the Child, arguably the foundation of children's universal right to participate. UNICEF, which had been formed in 1946 (UNICEF, 2022a) to deal with the after-effects on children of the Second World War, went on to draft the United Nations Convention on the Rights of the Child (UNCRC) in 1989 (UNICEF, 2022b). A thorough synopsis of the critical moments for children's liberty in the 20th century is provided by Martin Woodhead (Woodhead 2010) in the prologue to the *Handbook of Children and Young People's Participation* (Percy-Smith & Thomas 2010). The UNCRC was quickly adopted by most countries (the UK ratified in 1991), yet still to this day the emphasis of children's regulation and statute in most countries is on child protection and services to children: participation is rarely the focus. We can see through history that children were seen as possessions, then as the objects of state protection. The UNCRC positions children as at least participants and potentially as citizens. The starting point for a theoretical framework is children's right to participate, as enshrined within the UNCRC.

Participation as a Right

Participation is a human right and as such it covers the rights of all ages of humans, including infants, children, and adolescents. As Lansdown (2010) has pointed out, the significance of participation as a fundamental human right is that it is also a means by which people are enabled to realise other rights.

Under the UNCRC, children, which includes everyone aged 18 and under, are seen as human beings in their own right with childhood not just the precursor to becoming an adult. Research with children and young people demonstrates that they place a great value on being recognised as people with views, wishes, and feelings of their own and the ability to take part in decision making (Lansdown 2010). The dilemma for UNICEF at the time of drafting the UNCRC was how to grant children equal value while at the same time guaranteeing them the necessary protections. The dilemma was resolved in the four principles below that underpin the UNCRC:

- Non-Discrimination
- Best interests of the child
- The right to survival and development
- The views of the child.

The UNCRC is the most widely adopted human rights treaty in history and, as stated earlier, of the countries that have gone from ratification to developing child law most have focused more on the best interests of the child, protecting the child's development, and ensuring survival. While these are undoubtedly necessary, they emphasise protection rather than liberty. Non-discrimination and the right to express views are aspects of liberty, yet although non-discrimination is increasingly a feature of child law and policy, the inherent discrimination against children simply on the basis of their age is rarely mentioned. A very effective way to remove age discrimination for children is to promote liberty through participation.

The emphasis on the child's views, or 'voice', as defined in Article 12, has attracted criticism and, some suggest, has reached its limits (Johnson and West 2018). Indeed, even the emphasis on Article 12 may not always be helpful, since most of the Articles are inter-dependent. Lundy (2007:

932) has conceptualised Article 12 in relation to Articles 13, the right to information, 5, right to guidance by adults, 3, best interests of the child and 2, anti-discrimination. My position is that the voice of the child is central and is both the starting point and cornerstone of their participation. Participation is more than being heard, that would seem to be self-evident, but the emphasis in the UNCRC on children being heard is surely not accidental. When we speak of being heard we also mean being acknowledged, taken seriously, and being understood in a profound way so we can be accepted. The concept of voice may be taken in its broadest sense to include a diversity of participation experiences and practices.

Models of Participation

While there has been an absence of formal theory, the practice of children's participation has not occurred in a vacuum of ideas. Prior to the publication of Lundy's work, two very influential works have shaped children's participation since the latter half of the 20th century. Sherry Arnstein's (1969) ladder of citizen participation was for a time the only published guide available, so in the absence of anything more appropriate, leaders of children's participation adapted and adopted it. Sherry Arnstein worked in communities and was interested in citizen participation, which Arnstein equated to citizen power. In Arnstein's metaphorical ladder, the lower rungs denote no participation and a form of consultation that Arnstein calls tokenistic. As the rungs rise there is an increasing level of agency, control, and power. Arnstein was concerned with the redistribution of power, from the haves to the have-nots, explaining that 'participation without redistribution of power is an empty and frustrating process for the powerless' (Arnstein 1969: 216). Implicit in this thinking is the notion of social capital (Bourdieu 1986).

Roger Hart (1992), a child rights academic, at the time working for UNICEF, famously took Arnstein's idea of the ladder as a starting point and elaborated it specifically for children. Hart proposed that real participation does not begin to happen until rung six and above. This included 'adult initiated' approaches, where young people share decision making, 'child initiated and directed' and at the top of the ladder 'child initiated and shared with adults'. Hart illustrated these concepts with examples from international settings.

While Arnstein and Hart continue to be widely used and cited, there have been several other models of children's participation, notably those developed by Westhorp (1987), Rocha, (1997) and Shier, (2001).

Westhorp (1987) identified a six-stage spectrum, or continuum, of youth involvement. Unlike Arnstein's and Hart's ladders, the Westhorp continuum does not suggest that more or less control is more or less desirable. Instead, these options exist, and some will be more appropriate in certain situations than others. This creates the possibility of a choice of various approaches so that a range of young people across diverse settings can participate.

Rocha (1997) based their typology on the notion of empowerment, visualised as a ladder that moves from individual through to community participation, where each rung characterises power experiences. Shier (2001) offered a model consisting of five levels of participation. At each level, individuals and organisations demonstrate different degrees of commitment to the process of empowerment.

What all of the above models share is the representation of a successive and hierarchical process, which reflects 'a limited and fragmented conceptualisation of children's participation' (Malone and Hartung 2010: 27).

The popularity of participation models is an important consideration. They are visually impactful, simple to understand and can be straightforwardly applied in real life. It is perhaps not surprising that their popularity endures. Critics of participation models, however, find them simplistic and not reflective of complexity, as stated by Malone and Hartung (2010: 35):

> The ladder was a significant foundation for creating a field of study around children's participation. The weakness, then, is its focus on being a 'practical tool' rather than a theoretical framework; while it has served well for practitioners in the field, we believe there is now a need to develop a theory that will capture the complexities of that field.

Arnstein acknowledged the weaknesses in the ladder model, suggesting that real life is more complicated than a simple hierarchy. Arnstein had no wish to over-simplify, stating at the time:

> There is a critical difference between going through the empty ritual of participation and having the real power needed to affect the outcome of the process.
>
> (Arnstein 1969: 216)

Hart had the final word on their own model, reflecting over a decade later:

> I see the ladder lying in the long grass of an orchard at the end of the season. It has served its purpose. I look forward to the next season for I know there are so many different routes up through the branches and better ways to talk about how children can climb into meaningful, and shall we say fruitful, ways of working with others.
>
> (Hart 2008: 29)

A model that continues to gain momentum (Lundy 2007) proposes a new conceptualisation of UNCRC Article 12. Lundy's model comprises of four domains necessary for participation. These are neither sequential nor hierarchical, but can be viewed as cyclical. The domains are:

Space: Children must be given the opportunity to express a view.
Voice: Children must be facilitated to express their views.
Audience: The view must be listened to.
Influence: The view must be acted upon, as appropriate.

The Lundy model sets clear expectations of adults, who are the gate-keepers of the means by which children's participation can take place. It is in that sense still reflective of participation that is determined and led by adults.

Children and Adults Working Together

While adults have created our environmental, social, and political world, the children of today will live with the consequences.

> Children are a significant part of our communities, they have good ideas, and often they are not as constrained by, or invested in, institutions or practices in the same way that adults tend to be.
>
> (Johnson et al. 2020: 8)

Several contributors to this book were involved with the GIFT project (Great Involvement Future Thinking), which ran from 2012–2016 across England as part of the ambitious transformation programme for children's and young people's mental health services, children and young people's improving access to psychological therapies, otherwise known as CYPIAPT (for more information on CYPIAPT, see Chapter 14) (Anderson 2022).

The GIFT team initially comprised five adults, all of whom had worked extensively in children's and young people's mental health and allied services, and whose related expertise included advocacy, facilitation, change management and child-led evaluation and training. This combined participatory practice was given greater impetus by our determination to put participation on the mental health agenda, along with our impatience for change.

The remit from NHS England was to support local, regional, and national initiatives to establish and maintain children's participation in mental health services, with the goal of embedding participation into routine, everyday practice. The small adult team then set about recruiting young partners with lived experience of mental health difficulties and using services, to work alongside us. The aims were to model participation at the national level to lead by example those working in local services.

The experience of the GIFT team was that, with a few notable exceptions, children's participation was seen as a 'nice to have' rather than a 'must-do'. The team found that what was described as participation varied enormously, ranging from tokenistic, entirely adult-led activities all the way through to authentic practices in which children and adults worked in partnership or where children were taking the lead. The latter was considerably more rare, with most participation quite explicitly determined and led by adults (Anderson 2022). The literature emerging over the past several years confirms that the GIFT experience was typical; Farrar et al. (2010: 86) assert:

> The negative perceptions of adults and their expectation of what children and young people can achieve remain a significant barrier to the participation of children and young people universally.

Further claims are made by Johnson et al. (2020: 11):

> Despite strong evidence supporting the importance of including children's and young people's participation in development practice, work that genuinely consults with and incorporates children's views and understandings is still minimal.

While successive children's acts across the regions of the UK have rightly put the child at the centre of policy and thinking, the focus on protection rights has often been at the expense of children's liberty rights – which are exercised through participation. This has been interpreted as:

> a dichotomy between a paternalistic approach to children's participation (nurturance orientation) and an approach characterised by the promotion of autonomy (self-determination orientation).
> (Matthew et al. 2010: 121)

In contrast, when children are taken seriously by adults the participation between them can become transformative. This has been noted in cross-cultural studies where,

> In spite of the notorious existence of unequal power relationships between adults and young people, whenever the latter are taken into account, listened to and acknowledged in their ability to contribute to transforming their reality, they develop a feeling of self-confidence, they feel more secure and raise their self- esteem. The 'mutual trust' factor becomes essential to participation. This entails adult

facilitators putting trust in young people's abilities and ideas: and the youth trusting that the adults will indeed give them support and take them into account.

(Corona Caraveo et al. 2010)

Parents and Carers

Hart (1992) is clear that the family is the primary setting in which children can develop social responsibility and the agency required to participate. Hart does not view parental processes as one-way, asserting that parents can also learn from observing their children's competence. On this basis Hart argues for parents' and carers' active engagement in programmes of participation and sees the joint efforts of children and parents as potential catalysts for change, observing,

> Productive collaboration between young and old should be the core of any democratic society wishing to improve itself, while providing continuity between the past, present, and the future.
>
> (Hart 1992: 37)

Parental involvement is most often seen in school settings and since at least 2019 has been a focal point of inspections by the Office for Standards in Education, Children's Services and Skills (OFSTED), in which inspectors assess 'whether leaders seek to engage parents and their community thoughtfully and positively in a way that supports pupils' education' (OFSTED 2019: 64).

Campaigning and training organisation, Just Add Parents (2022) provides a timeline of parental involvement in education for over 50 years. They illustrate the shifts in emphasis as both governments and pedagogical thinking have changed, claiming that since around 1970 parental involvement has more than doubled in intensity.

Outside of schools, parent and carer involvement is more patchy and when compared with the proliferation of children's participation activities, it perhaps reinforces again the significance of the UNCRC. While Article 5 provides for parental provision of direction and guidance according to children's developmental stages, the focus of the other articles is necessarily on children.

The major interest of the GIFT project was children's participation and, particularly at the national level where older young people were involved in partnership working with adults on policy and strategy, this did not readily involve parents and carers. Where GIFT supported the greatest volume of activity though was in participation communities connected to children's services and here it was more common to find parents and carers participating alongside children. Where very young children were participating the involvement of a parent or carer was often a necessity. Given that the views and interests of parents/carers, while they may overlap, will often be different from those of children, we found the most successful initiatives were those that separated the two groups so that each could pursue their own agenda, perhaps coming together at a later point. Reconciling the different processes and outcomes required skilled facilitation and where this happened the outcomes were positive. Having children try to participate in situations where their own parent or carer was present was often found to be counter-productive and not helpful for either the children or the adults.

Levels of Participation

At the micro-level, participation can work at the smallest levels of inter-action, for instance an individual child or young person can participate in decisions about their own life. In mental health services this might be by setting goals in partnership with the therapist and being instrumental in assessing or measuring their achievement of the goals. Young people in social care can participate in their case reviews and other significant meetings so that decisions about them are made with them. Whenever a child or young person is using a service, there is opportunity for their participation at the micro-level.

When children and young people participate in groups, this is known as participating at the meso-level. Participation groups, whether in person, digital, or hybrid, have been a popular feature of forward-looking services for children for many years. At the meso-level it is possible for participation to impact more people and processes than at the micro level. It promotes social change and informal peer support and is easier for young people to take a leadership role than individual participation. Participation at the meso level often has a transformative focus, whether aimed within a service or organisation, across a locality, or within a neighbourhood.

Large-scale change is possible when young people participate at the macro-level, joining with adults in teams and groups where decisions are made about wide-ranging policy and processes. Macro-level participation may take place in national or sometimes international contexts.

In the transformation programme that GIFT was part of, participation at the micro-level took place when children were involved in goal setting and self-assessing the outcomes of mental health interventions. This required changes to practice for many mental health professionals and was supported by resources and training. The GIFT team supported meso-level participation throughout the regions and localities, facilitating local events, hosting master classes, and sharing learning through the dissemination of resources and bringing participation people together online. A distinctive element of GIFT was the recruitment of young advisors, who were trained and supported to take part in national decision making and policy groups, in some cases taking over the chairing or leadership of the event. The national young advisors also led workshops, spoke at professionals' meetings, created resources, and delivered their own national conference.

Impact and Benefits of Participation

The recent REJUVENATE (Johnson et al. 2020) project conducted a scoping of practitioner and academic literature, resulting in a literature review matrix and a typology of existing approaches, finding that,

> participatory development work with children has significant instrumental, conceptual, capacity-building, and connectivity benefits. Instrumental impact relates to a project influencing the development of policy, practice or service provision, shaping legislation, or altering behaviour; conceptual impact happens when a project contributes to the understanding of policy issues, or reframing debates; capacity-building impact relates to technical and personal skill development; and connectivity to increased relationships, partnerships and networks that can support impact.
>
> (Johnson et al. 2020: 27)

This resonates with my own experiences and relates in many ways to the '5 ways to wellbeing' (Aked et al. 2008), which provides evidence for the benefits to mental health of being active, connecting socially, continuously learning, taking notice, and giving to others. Since the five ways are also typical of participation activities, it helps to explain the observation that participation in GIFT seemed to result in improved mental health for the young people who worked alongside the adults. These findings are also supported by work conducted in a Headspace service in Australia (Coates and Howe 2014) as well as in the literature around mental health and participation in adults (Fletcher and Sarkar 2013) and is explored in further chapters of this book.

What Johnson et al. (2020) refer to above as instrumental benefits might also be called having influence on decision making, which has been described as potentially transformative of adult–child relations (Mason and Bolzan 2010: 129). The references to both capacity building and connectivity to others point to a benefit of participation, especially at the meso and macro levels, being the development of social capital. This is significant: social capital is a sociological concept usually associated with Pierre Bourdieu (1986), which helps to explain structural advantages and disadvantages affecting people from different social groups. Generally, those children from more privileged backgrounds have high social capital, which gives them the advantage over their peers. A lack of social capital is exacerbated when children and young people are in situations that make them vulnerable, and included in this are situations in which services are used, such as mental health, special education, or youth justice (see Morrow 2017).

> Unlike human capital, which focuses on the individuals' abilities, and economic capital, which measures possession, social capital addresses the networks and ties, in which individuals are woven in. Being a member of a network gives you an advantage, as you gain information, support, access and trust. Through these aspects, social capital can improve one's life satisfaction and well-being.
>
> (Klocke and Studmüller 2018: 1169)

Summary

The foregoing has provided an overview of recent developments in the field of children's participation, a synopsis of literature, and lived experience. This synopsis illustrates the requirement for a theory of children's and young people's participation and it is clear that such a theory needs to be sufficiently robust to stand up against critiques of existing models and recent practice.

The preceding review has shown that a theory of children's participation will need to take account of constructions of childhood and the status of children and their participation. Children must be understood as capable young citizens, with adults as enablers or supporters, rather than controllers. The theory should be founded upon universal children's rights and emphasise both liberty and choice.

The rigour required to develop this theory is through the systematic reasoning of multiple perspectives, forming a dialectical theoretical framework. The framework is offered as a foundation for theory.

Towards a Theory of Children's and Young People's Participation: A Framework

This proposed framework applies to children's and young people's participation in all matters affecting them, applying specifically, but not restrictively, to the services they use. These services may be in a myriad of settings across health, education, social care, and youth justice.

In developing a theory of children's participation, the framework may be used minimally as a checklist to ensure that all the salient components are included. More fully the framework can be employed to invoke searching questions about the status of children and the nature of participation, imbuing meaning into the act of participating and identifying the beneficial outcomes for individuals, organisations, and wider society.

The Framework

Children means infants, children, and young people from birth to 25.

- This includes all children, by right, regardless of any characteristic. Age in itself is not a barrier to a child's ability to participate.
- Defining the upper end of childhood as 25 enables inclusion and diversity.
- Children are citizens in their own right and not simply the adults of the future.
- Children are capable of leading participation for children.
- Some children need support from others to participate.

Children's participation happens when in any area affecting them:

- Children's voices are heard.
- Children's views, wishes, and feelings influence decision making.
- Children have agency.

Children's participation is founded on universal rights.

- Starting with human rights, which apply to all ages of humans.
- Specifically focused on children's rights contained within the UNCRC – primarily Article 12, but in the context of the interdependency of all the Articles.
- Responsibility for ensuring those rights are upheld lies ultimately with the government.

Children's participation is supported by enabling adults.

- Adults' roles are to facilitate the participation both by preparing themselves to listen and respond appropriately and to help children learn new skills through coaching, mentoring, and modelling.
- In the first instance, adults will create enabling environments for participation that take account of children's age and circumstances.
- Adults will in turn be supported by children to develop skills that promote participation.

Children's participation is always inclusive.

- Children of all ages, abilities, and backgrounds are able to participate.

- Environments are adapted to enable inclusive participation.
- Inclusive participation acknowledges power differences and works towards equal partnership between the people of all ages who are participating.

The theory of children's participation is applied to practice.

- The practice of children's participation can be both individual and collective.
- Participation occurs at all levels – micro, meso and macro.
- These levels are not hierarchical but are situational.

The theory and practice of children's participation have purpose.

- Participation leads to change and is transformational not transactional.
- Participation produces beneficial outcomes.
- Those leading or facilitating participation are accountable to the participating children for supporting or enabling the achievement of beneficial outcomes.

The beneficial outcomes to children of participation are:

- Changes and improvements to policy and processes that affect them directly or indirectly.
- Increased self-esteem, self-confidence, self-efficacy.
- Greater social connections and personal relationships.
- Increased skills and knowledge.
- Greater social capital.

There can be little doubt that children's and young people's participation has value and meaning, producing positive outcomes. Additionally, these attributes need to be captured and articulated to serve both as a guide for practice and the foundation for research.

Children's and young people's participation is an unstoppable force: the time for a theory of children's and young people's participation is surely now.

References

Aked, J., Marks, N., Cordon, C. & Thompson, S. (2008). *A Report Presented to the Foresight Project on Communicating the Evidence Base for Improving People's Well-being*. Centre for well-being.

Alderson, P., Sutcliffe, K. & Curtis, K. (2006). Children's competence to consent to medical treatment. *The Hastings Center Report*, 36 (6) 25–34.

Arnstein, S. (1969). A ladder of citizen participation. *Journal of the American Institute of Planners* 35 (4). https://www.tandfonline.com/doi/pdf/10.1080/01944366908977225.

Bourdieu, P. (1986). The forms of capital. In Richardson, J.G., Ed., (1986). *Handbook of Theory and Research for the Sociology of Education.* Greenwood Press: New York, 241–258.

Casey, B. J., Jones, R. M. & Hare, T. A. (2008). The adolescent brain. *Annals of the New York Academy of Sciences*, 1124, 111–126. https://doi.org/10.1196/anna ls.1440.010.

Cherry, K. (2022). Piaget's 4 stages of cognitive development explained: Background and key concepts of Piaget's theory. Updated on May 02, 2022. https://www.verywellmind.com/piagets-stages-of-cognitive-development-2795457.

Cherry, K. (2021). Erik Erikson's stages of psychosocial development. Updated on July 18, 2021. https://www.verywellmind.com/erik-eriksons-stages-of-psychoso cial-development-2795740.

Coates, D. & Howe, D. (2014). The importance and benefits of youth participation in mental health settings from the perspective of the Headspace Gosford Youth Alliance in Australia. *Children and Youth Services Review*, 46, 294–299.

Corona Caraveo, Y., Pérez, C. & and Hernández, J. (2010). Youth participation in indigenous traditional communities, in Percy-Smith, B., & Thomas, N., Eds. (2010). *A Handbook of Children and Young People's Participation: Perspectives from Theory and Practice.* Routledge: Abingdon.

Farrar, F., Ghannam, T., Manning, J. & Munroe, E. (2010). Commentary 1, in Percy-Smith, B., & Thomas, N., Eds. (2010). *A Handbook of Children and Young People's Participation: Perspectives from Theory and Practice.* Routledge: Abingdon.

Fletcher, D. & Sarkar, M. (2013). Psychological resilience: A review and critique of definitions, concepts, and theory. *European Psychologist* 18, 12–23.

Anderson, Y. (2022). *GIFT Guide to Sustaining Participation: Great Involvement Future Thinking.* Kindle Edition. https://www.amazon.co.uk/dp/B09XYNSQXG.

Hart, R. (1992). Children's participation: From tokenism to citizenship. UNICEF. https://www.unicef-irc.org/publications/pdf.

Hart, R. (2008). *Stepping Back from 'The Ladder': Reflections on a Model of Participatory Work with Children in Participation and Learning*, 2008, 19–31.

Johnson, V. & West, A. (2018). *Children's Participation in Global Contexts Going Beyond Voice.* Routledge: Abingdon.

Johnson, V., Lewin, T. & Cannon, M. (2020). *Learning from a Living Archive: Rejuvenating Child and Youth Rights and Participation*, REJUVENATE Working Paper 1.

Just Add Parents (2022). https://justaddparents.co.uk/improve-parent-communica tion/parent-involvement-brief-history-policy-intervention.

Klocke, A. & Stadtmüller, S. (2017). Social capital in the health development of children. *European University Institute Department of Political and Social Sciences. Child Ind Res* (2019) 12, 1167–1185.

Lansdown, G. (2010). The realisation of children's participation rights: Critical reflections, in Percy-Smith, B., & Thomas, N., Eds. (2010). *A Handbook of Children and Young People's Participation: Perspectives from Theory and Practice.* Routledge: Abingdon.

Leguina, A. & Miles, A. (2017). Fields of participation and lifestyle in England: Revealing the regional dimension from a reanalysis of the Taking Part Survey using Multiple Factor Analysis, *Cultural Trends* 26(1), 4–17.

Lundy, L. (2007). Voice' is not enough: Conceptualising Article 12 of the United Nations Convention on the Rights of the Child. *British Educational Research Journal* 33(6), 927–942.

Malone, K. & and Hartung, C. (2010). Challenges of participatory practice with children, in Percy-Smith, B., & Thomas, N., Eds. (2010). *A Handbook of Children and Young People's Participation: Perspectives from Theory and Practice.* Routledge: Abingdon.

Mason, J. & Bolzan, N. (2010). Questioning understandings of children's participation: Applying a cross-cultural lens, in Percy-Smith, B., & Thomas, N., Eds. (2010). *A Handbook of Children and Young People's Participation: Perspectives from Theory and Practice.* Routledge: Abingdon.

Matthew, A., Martelli, A., & Bertozzi, R. *et al.* (2010). Commentary 2 – Reflections on the participation of particular groups, in *A Handbook of Children and Young People's Participation.* Routledge: Abingdon.

Morrow, V. (2017). Conceptualising social capital in relation to the well-being of children and young people: A critical review. *The Sociological Review* June 2008, 744–761.

OFSTED (2019). *Schools Inspection Handbook.* Retrieved from School Inspection Handbook (https://www.gov.uk/government/publications/school-inspection-handbook-eif/school-inspection-handbook#evaluating-leadership-and-management).

Percy-Smith, B. & Thomas, N. Eds. (2010). *A Handbook of Children and Young People's Participation: Perspectives from Theory and Practice.* Routledge: Abingdon.

Rocha, E. (1997). A ladder of empowerment. *Journal of Planning, Education and Research*, 17, 31–44.

Shier, H. (2001). Pathways to participation: openings, opportunities and obligations: a new model for enhancing children's participation in decision-making, in line with article 12.1 of the United Nations Convention on the Rights of the Child. *Children & Society*, 15(2), 107–117.

Tierney, A. L. & Nelson, C. A. 3rd (2009). Brain development and the role of experience in the early years. *Zero to Three*, 30(2), 9–13.

UNICEF (2022a). https://www.unicef.org/history.

UNICEF (2022b). https://www.unicef.org.uk/what-we-do/un-convention-child-rights/.

Westhorp, G. (1987). *Planning for Youth Participation: A Resource Kit.* Adelaide: Youth Sector Training Council of South Australia.

Woodhead, M. (2010). Foreword, in Percy-Smith, B. & Thomas, N. Eds. (2010). *A Handbook of Children and Young People's Participation: Perspectives from Theory and Practice.* Routledge: Abingdon.

Chapter 3

Tokensim Versus Meaningful Engagement

Leanne Walker (She/They)

Introduction

I am writing this chapter from the perspective of someone with lived experience of mental health difficulties, who has been involved in a breadth of participation work across children and young people's (CYPs) mental health and beyond for the last near decade. I have experienced a range of work spanning from personally feeling 'tokenistic', like a 'tick box exercise', to 'genuine', and 'truly collaborative'. I have worked with and observed many others who describe participation work in similar ways. I have witnessed different people feel both happy and unhappy within the same piece of work described as participation, with some people happy to be in the space and others wanting clearer roles, actions, and outcomes. Literature widely evidences that participation can occur across healthcare, yet for many reasons it does not happen (Ocloo and Matthews 2016: 626), and in other instances it is branded as 'tokenistic' or other words to the same effect including, 'tokenism', 'token gesture' and a 'tick box'. This chapter seeks to explore what is behind these commonly heard phrases. What is really meant by tokenism within CYPs participation? Is it as simple as 'tokenistic' participation at one end of a scale and 'meaningful engagement' at the other? This chapter will be an exploration based on literature and lived experiences.

A Note

In this chapter, when discussing involvement in participation or involvement of people with lived experience, I am referring to children and young people (CYP) with experience of mental health difficulties and parents, carers, or family members with experience of supporting a child or young person with mental health difficulties across a range of mental health settings.

It is also important to note, that due to the often negative connotations of the word tokenism, this chapter does not intend to point fingers of blame or otherwise. Tokenism is often seen as incorrect or engagement 'gone wrong'

DOI: 10.4324/9781003288800-3

(Majid 2020: 1610), where phrases such as 'tokenistic participation', are often used to refer to practice seen as less than good enough (Lundy 2018: 2).

It does however, seek to explore tokenism in CYPs mental health, digging deeper under what is meant by it, and acknowledge that often those in healthcare systems have a commitment to involving those with lived experiences, but feel they do not know how to or have knowledge gaps (Ocloo and Matthews 2016: 626). It also explores meaningful participation and some of the obstacles or aspects to be worked through. By doing so, it hopes to stoke reflection, changes in practice, and learning for those wanting to do participation within CYPs mental health settings.

What Exactly is Tokenism? Exploring Defining/Conceptualising Tokenism

Tokenism as 'Non-participation'

Within the literature 'tokenism' is often used or cited with little explanation as to what it actually means, apart from indicating it is something negative. It is often dropped in with the assumption that what it is, is understood. Often it is used to describe a situation where participation has been attempted but for whatever reason it was not truly genuine, did not feel like or was not observed by others as participation, or felt like a misplaced go at participation.

When exploring tokenism, Hart's (1992) Ladder of Participation (based on Arnstein 1969) cannot be ignored. Tokenism on Hart's ladder appears as rung 3 within the same bracket as 'non-participation' (Hart 1992: 8). Also in this bracket sits 'Manipulation' and 'Decoration' (Hart 1992: 8). Tokenism as 'non-participation' is seen to occur when CYP are given the opportunity to share their views, but are given limited flexibility for how to express them and which parts to share (Hart 1992: 8–10).

Maybe, it looked like participation was attempted, as such, but actually ended up not really being participation at all. For example, someone may be asked only to share a certain part of what they wanted to, or have to share their views in a certain way, which does not suit the person. Or perhaps the participation opportunity seeking views of CYP was in the daytime, when most CYP are at school, meaning who could take part was limited and not representative.

Questions then arise including, is it still tokenism if someone had genuinely wanted to, and set out to, do meaningful participation well, but for whatever reason (for example, knowledge gaps), it did not happen as such? Does it make a difference to participation being described as tokenistic, if the participation space has been created out of a genuine, true want for CYP and parents and carers to participate, yet it did not turn out that way? Or, is tokenism related to participation spaces created out of something other than genuine intent? For example, because someone needs to, policy indicates they should, or have been told to, or otherwise. So has 'non-participation' (Hart 1992: 8) occurred due to a misplaced genuine intent? And is that the same as or different to tokenistic participation?

When I was in a CYPs mental health service participation group, working with clinical members of staff, you could feel their genuine interest, want, and intent to do meaningful participation well. This was felt through their actions, words, and body language. Yet, some of the blockers to the work we wanted to achieve together came from more senior colleagues, such as managers and those above, who did not understand what it was we were trying to do, or were not making time for us or even being engaged. This did not feel tokenistic in the participation group space because it felt like intent in the 'room' was genuine, but it felt tokenistic when thinking about those more senior/the wider context. At the time, it did not always feel that they were listening or genuinely interested in what we were doing or saying. This may have been through miscommunication or other explanations, but it still existed as a collective feeling in that local-level participation group space and created this dual dynamic of genuine participation and tokenism. It is important to have that broader awareness of the context in understanding participation, which comes to be described as tokenistic.

Context

There are also physical, practical, and emotional elements to be considered and explored when understanding participation described as tokenistic. Has what it means to 'do participation' been considered, such as awareness of meeting times and then who can participate, having a safe physical space, and any emotional support that might be needed. Or are there knowledge gaps that have led to the practise described as tokenistic? Hahn et al. (2017: 291) suggest people can unintentionally participate in tokenism through being unaware of what actual engagement is. Warming (2011: 131) suggests that good intent alone is not enough for participation to not be tokenistic and other external factors are also important. Someone can have intent to do genuine participation in a way not experienced as tokenistic, have the skill and knowledge to do so, but it is also dependant on a range of factors such as the culture and politics of the service they are working in, which may not be conducive with what is to be done (Warming 2011: 131).

Culture

Literature also evidences culture to be important in tokenism. Macgregor (2022: 158), when discussing participation in mental health tribunal processes, highlights the importance of a shift in culture if participation is not to be experienced in a tokenistic way. The culture of participation and the way it is viewed is important so it is not seen as an 'add on' or a nice, additional extra rather than fundamental and integral across the service or space. It is also suggested that tokenism occurs when culture is only listening to voices who bring a perspective that supports existing perspectives (Majid 2020: 1611). This could be continuing to head in this direction, even though it has been voiced by a lived-experience majority to be an incorrect direction. If participation is not embedded into culture and seen as a 'must do', perhaps it then can be tokenistic. For further discussion on culture change see Chapter 14.

For Appearance Only?

In other literature, tokenism is seen as a practice where only minimal effort, often referred to as 'symbolic effort' is put into involving lived experiences (Hahn et al. 2017: 290). Also along these lines, tokenism in CYPs participation has also been referred to as 'lip service', 'fostering resentment in service users' (Barrett 2010: 80), supporting the notion that tokenism is seen as wrong (Majid 2020: 1611). For example, tokenism can be the act of agreeing something with CYP or parents and carers, but with no actual real action attached, or maybe a decision has already been made and voices of support are only being sought in order to go ahead, so only on appearance does it look like wanted actions are happening and lived experience is being heard and acted upon. The idea that tokenism is around doing something for appearances only, leaving people with lived experience(s) unhappy, is captured in Elizabeth's experience as a young person:

> I have an example which to me is the definition of tokenism. I was asked to sit on a conference panel and give a presentation about my experiences using mental health services. We were selected by the organisers and ended up being all female with only one of five of us being from a BIPOC (Black, Indigenous and People of Colour) background even though our service is in a very multicultural area. We weren't given chance to talk with other young people about the topic, and the presentation had already been written for us! It felt like we were just there for show. It was a waste of my time and I don't feel like I got to make a difference.
>
> Elizabeth

Tokenism as a Feeling

The lived experience example above, draws out an important point that is yet to be considered here when exploring conceptualising tokenism, suggesting tokenism in participation is about a feeling, that it is as much about how the participation space feels to an individual. Namely it becomes tokenistic when it leaves people with negative feelings. This certainly chimes with my own lived experience, when I have felt unheard, felt not listened to, felt like I was there just to evidence that lived experience had been considered. It left me with feelings I would describe as negative (such as frustration, sadness and anger). It was these experiences that I would often then describe as tokenistic, as being there as a token or ticking a box; my opinion was never going to be truly heard, considered or acted upon, whatever I did. This was regardless of expression of intent of those who had coordinated the participation, in terms of whether they spoke about really wanting to involve those with lived experience or not. If it *felt* like intent was not genuine and actions did not match words, then I experienced it as tokenism. This suggests tokenism in participation cannot be conceptualised without considering how those participating feel about it.

Exploring Further

Looking at broader definitions, The Cambridge Dictionary (2022) defines tokenism as:

> something that a person or organization does that seems to support or help a group of people who are treated unfairly in society. Such as giving a member of that group an important or public position, but which is not meant to make changes that would help that group of people in a lasting way.

The difference in angle here is that tokenism applies to 'people who are treated unfairly in society' (Cambridge Dictionary 2022), suggesting it is merely to create the illusion of change rather than actual change. Fleming (2013: 486) discusses tokenism in participation and also highlights 'much participation is based on the more powerful inviting the less powerful'. Combined, this thinking draws out that perhaps power and privilege cannot be ignored when conceptualising tokenism. Majid (2020: 1611) states,

> Health service organizations are especially susceptible to tokenism because of the natural power differences that exist between patients and health care professionals.

Looking historically, this power imbalance was entrenched in history where the relationship between people accessing services and those working in services was largely paternalistic. Whereby medical treatments were administered or withheld based purely on the perceived medical benefit (Pollard 1993). This power imbalance was particularly strong in mental health services with the power to segregate and confine, where during the mid-17th century those deemed to have a 'mental illness' were systematically and extensively confined (Foucault 1988).

In more recent history, it is still documented that there exists power imbalances between those accessing services and those working within them (Strickler 2009; Hitchen et al. 2011; Aoki 2020). Is tokenism an extension (or consequence) of this history?

As someone with lived experience of being involved in participation in CYPs mental health services, power was never spoken about, but it was still experienced. Ultimately, it was the service that had the power to stop or start any idea we had as a participation group. There were things we wanted to do and achieve but did not have the authority, budget or go ahead from managers and senior leaderships, which prevented us moving forward and vice versa. Of course, many things were given the go ahead and many things we could do, the key here was that it was largely in the control of others and we were aware of this. Eventually we carried out our own fundraising activities so we could have our own small budget, giving us more power and control over what we wanted to do as a participation group. This is why power should also be included when defining tokenism in CYP/parent and carer participation. However, it also suggests tokenism can be used as a stepping-stone to other forms of engagement. In my example, not being able to do what we felt would be of benefit and fuelled us to find other means to go forward. This was Lundy's (2018: 8) conclusion stating 'children gave examples of how tokenistic responses galvanised them into further action'.

Privilege

On the other hand if 'people who are treated unfairly in society' (Cambridge Dictionary 2022), are not even around the metaphorical table, this circles back to participation not really happening at all. Is it tokenism when attempts are not made to include a broad range of perspectives? For example, when the participation event is 1pm on Wednesday when most people are at school or work, only those with the privilege to take time off are able to engage and take part. Someone may be chosen as they share a positive view of the participation event, which supports existing views, rather than a critical one (Hart 1992). Or people with lived experience are not representative of the local population. It is documented that disabled communities, the homeless population, and those more likely to 'challenge the system' are among those most often excluded (Ocloo and Matthews 2016: 628) or are sometimes invited, but genuinely not supported to over-come barriers to involvement making it difficult or impossible to participate.

Are those decisions around who is invited to participate, when they are invited, and how they are invited made consciously or unconsciously? Therefore, should unconscious bias also be considered when conceptualising what tokenism is?

I have been involved in a lot of participation work where it has been known that voices are missing from the room, but it has been expressed that it is 'too hard' and 'easier' to do participation with the people who come forward themselves. I have also been involved in examples of people being completely unaware of diversity of lived experience and therefore not even knowingly excluding people. Is it tokenism in participation when people put minimal effort into who is being listened to and who is not, whether they do this consciously or unconsciously? This perhaps links back to Hahn's et al. (2017: 290) 'symbolic effort'. It is therefore important that those doing participation are educated around unconscious bias and turning unconscious bias into conscious actions around what can be done to ensure a breadth of lived experience inclusion.

Is it all Bad?

In exploring literature and lived experiences so far, tokenism has been largely associated with negative experiences, as something that is bad and not what the mental health field should be doing, but when trying to define tokenism, it is important to question whether tokenism is all bad. Lundy (2018: 14) suggests that tokenism can be used as a means 'to do nothing at all'. For example 'I don't want involvement of lived experiences to be tokenistic, so I won't even try'. This demonstrates a lack of will/want/resources to put in the effort to do meaningful participation. But, is that worse than not even trying at all? With this, Lundy (2018: 15) concludes tokenistic practise to be far from ideal, but a starting point to build from is better than doing nothing at all.

It is also acknowledged that not all CYP, parents, and carers want to participate in all the ways that someone can participate across the mental health field (Barrett 2010: 80). Participating in some way may feel better than not participating at all and therefore perhaps may become a positive experience. My own lived experience example, above, highlights how the participation space evolved. This circles back to tokenism as a feeling and how someone, as an individual, interprets what has happened, how it feels, and what sits well for them. Someone may experience something as tokenistic, which another person may not.

A Summary

This look into what is meant by the word tokenism has evidenced that there are a lot of factors that are captured by the use of one simple word.

To bring them all together would suggest tokenism to be mostly seen as something negative. Yet it can also be an opportunity to grow from, where people with lived experience, sometimes only representing certain experiences/demographics, are consciously or unconsciously selected or invited to participate by those with more power and privilege. Where people cannot always share their genuine thoughts/feelings through a means/space and time that suits all, there can perhaps be a lack of genuine intent or culture to do participation. This therefore has resulted in not dispelling/or thinking through barriers, which may not be through lack of want, but may be down to wider factors, leaving those participating, or others in the same space, with negative feelings.

The Risks of Tokenism

Elizabeth's experience below highlights the feelings of tokenism that can also occur within participation in own care:

> When my worker explained to me the options for support I could receive, they were very pushy about wanting me to go for family therapy. I didn't feel like I needed family therapy, my family are very supportive and understanding. It was like here are your choices but I didn't really have a choice. Other options like CBT [Cognitive Behavioural Therapy] (which I eventually had) weren't properly talked about, and I felt like there was nothing out there to help me. It made me feel like I had no control over what happened to me. Plus my [other] worker agreed I didn't need it [family therapy].
>
> Elizabeth

Elizabeth's worker presented choice, but ultimately guided Elizabeth into what they thought was right. This goes against the notion of shared decision making, the idea that choices should be presented to those accessing services and decisions made collaboratively (Hayes et al. 2018). Elizabeth did not feel this happened and that what they did not want was pushed. This highlights the power imbalance in tokenistic participation in care and perhaps is also a risk to the therapeutic relationship, which is evidenced as 'key' to progress (Mercer et al. 2015: 80). The establishment of a therapeutic relationship between those accessing services and those using them can be an important element to progress (Walker 2020: 22). Making meaningful participation in one's own care important.

Tokenistic participation can also be used to legitimise decision making that has already taken place instead of being open to new ideas and ways of thinking (Farrington 2016: 370). At the heart of it, this suggests tokenism threatens the democratic accountability of mental health systems. Patient safety scandals in the UK called for greater participation to prevent further serious failings. For example, the Bristol Inquiry high-lighted 'a failure to put patients at the centre of care' (Department of Health 2002: 1). With a lack of patient and carer involvement depriving the hospital of important information, leaving patients and parents and carers feeling 'a sense of bewilderment' and exclusion (The Bristol Royal Infirmary Inquiry 2001: 400).

Recommendations from The Bristol Royal Infirmary Inquiry (2001: 456–457) included:

- 'The involvement of the public in the NHS must be embedded in its structures: the perspectives of patients and of the public must be heard and taken into account wherever decisions ... are made'.
- 'The public's involvement in the NHS should particularly be focused on the development and planning of healthcare services and on the operation and delivery of healthcare services, including the regulation of safety and quality, the competence of healthcare professionals, and the protection of vulnerable groups.
- 'The process of public involvement must be properly supported, through for example, the provision of training and guidance'.
- 'Primary care trusts ... must make efforts systematically to gather views and feedback from patients'.

Meaningful Engagement

The next half of this chapter shall explore some of the considerations that it may be useful to work through and reflect on before undertaking par-ticipation activities, in order to move away from participation described as tokenistic and towards participation described as meaningful.

It will not be exhaustive or extensive, but rather a guide. Obviously consideration needs to be given to individual circumstances and situations and suggestions may need to be adapted to fit those. It will be split into sections and aims to offer learning and insight from the perspective of having been involved in various participation spaces and roles.

Time and Support

Participation takes time to do. It can sometimes be better to do a smaller/ 'simpler' thing well, than take on something bigger if there is not the time to do it meaningfully. If there are deadlines and timescales, then acknowledging, recognising, and sharing this is important. If a participa-tion activity is rushed through without explanation of the timeframes that need to be met, this can lead to it feeling tokenistic as people are not given the space and time needed to work on something and do not know why it is being rushed. Generally, if explained to those participating that there are timescales and deadlines, people tend to understand that time pressures exist and systems do work to deadlines.

As well as requiring actual time to do participation, it also requires a broader time commitment. This includes time to support people to be involved both practically and emotionally, these aspects cannot be overlooked. For example, if asking someone with lived experience to participate in a meeting, is there time to meet beforehand and after in a pre-meet and de-brief to provide a space to answer questions, make sure everyone is okay and has what they need? Is there an agenda shared in advance so people can make an informed choice as to whether they want to be involved in discussions around those topics? Is there an opportunity to feed into the agenda?

Another example I come across often, in terms of time, is a clinical member of staff asking to come to a lived experience meeting to ask for feedback on a project. When asked how much time they would like on the agenda, the required allotment of time can be '10–15' minutes. In practice this ends up being the person coming, talking for ten minutes explaining in brief what they are doing, and leaving. Often those in the space do not have the right depth of information to be able to digest it, are not given enough time to explore what they are being asked about/do not know/are not told what happens after they have provided input, making it feel tokenistic. If there is a genuine want to have lived experience input, there needs to be adequate time to do so and time to revise the project/direction if the lived experience input indicates this. It is also important to close the feedback loop, and go back to those who participated and share what happened/what was the outcome of their input, even if that feedback is 'we tried to do X and we couldn't because...'

Resources

To put in adequate time to do participation requires resources – people are a resource. Often this requires it to be in a job description so enough time can be put into doing it meaningfully. This obviously requires funding and an argument for participation. I have come across examples where it is additional to people's day jobs (not job planned) and therefore the first thing to drop off when competing priorities come along. I have also heard many examples where a participation worker has been funded, which increases time capacity and resource, but often the worker is employed in isolation or without being attached to a team. I have also known situations where Participation Workers have had unclear structures around line management and supervision. This isolation can create a sense of disconnect from the wider service/team and it is viewed as their responsibility to do participation, rather than it being everyone's responsibility and what the whole team or service should be working towards. It is important to think about wider structures and support for people in isolated roles.

Funding/a budget will also need to be identified in order to do any work needed. For example, if there is a participation group which has found a gap in service resource and wants to develop something they will likely need funds to do this. Funds may also be needed for practical aspects such as a meeting space and refreshments. Thought might also need to be given to reimbursing people for their time and any travel expense. In experience, paying people for their time adds to feelings of being valued for knowledge, skills, and experience brought, building on the sense of meaningful participation.

Wider Support

When aiming to do meaningful participation considering wider structures is important. For example if you are paying people's expenses, is the expense process known, accessible, and timely? I have many personal lived experiences of having to endlessly chase payments in a way that would not be tolerated or acceptable to permanent staff on the payroll. It also can unintentionally exclude people from taking part. For example, if someone is living paycheque to paycheque and reliant on knowing when income will be received, they may not be able to spend time involved in something in which they do not reliably know when expenses will be paid. Wider support involves looking at the wider system, what is in place already and what needs to be put in place.

In terms of wider support and structure is there also a known and active chain or route of escalation and support if needed such as managers, decision makers, and budget holders that can support projects and work, release funds, arrange wider meetings, and take ideas elsewhere. It is important to have this when asking people to come up with ideas and projects for improvement. There needs to be the actual means to make these happen so it does not feel tokenistic.

Consideration should also be given to emotional support. Often people in lived experience participation spaces are asked to talk about really difficult times and share really difficult things. Conceptualising tokenism as a feeling suggests the consideration of how those participating are feeling, checking in and adjusting accordingly is important. But also awareness and recognition that it can be emotionally hard and people may need emotional support to participate.

Being Mindful of Personal Thoughts and Feelings

Some services use outcome measurement tools to support participation in an individual's own care. But without the right language around such tools, they can become tokenistic. I have found that sometimes personal thoughts and feelings influence clinicians' own language in reference to these. Elizabeth also evidences this:

> My [clinician] always used to ask me to rate the session at the end saying it was something we just had to do. It felt really pointless. It was just a form I had to fill out and honestly? I just ticked boxes and I'm not even sure what it was used for.
>
> Elizabeth

As someone with lived experience, I have positive and negative personal experience of outcome measures being used to facilitate participation and collaboration in my own care. When presented as 'sorry but the service requires me to ask you to fill these out', I have felt I should not care about them either and that they clearly do not mean a lot anyway. This then created this feeling of tokenism and ticking a box. The language used by the mental health worker and whether they truly believe in them and value them as tools, can make those accessing services see the value in them also. When used meaningfully, CYP report 'positive experiences' (Law et al. 2015: 34), as opposed to the more tokenistic. Sometimes this requires clinicians to be mindful of their own thoughts and feelings and not assume what CYP will think about such tools.

Making Assumptions

We all make assumptions about different things and it is important we are aware of this when working in mental health (Willig 2019). I have often heard phrases such as 'CYP would not be interested in this', 'this is boring', or 'we will only show them the interesting parts'. Yet, as humans we have such vast and differing interests, there is sure to be someone out there with an interest in what we personally find boring. We can make assumptions of others interests based on our own interest and opinion on something. This can sometimes lead to not sharing all the information or the whole picture as it is deemed 'boring' or 'uninteresting'. There can also be assumptions around the information being too complex or hard to understand.

I have experienced many situations where CYP and parents and carers have been asked to participate in something, but information has been omitted for being 'too complex'. This has meant people could not truly participate as they did not have the level of information required. Sometimes a step back is needed to question whether personal feelings on something are leading to making assumptions about others.

Language

At times, it can feel like the mental health field has created its own language with all the shortened words, terms, acronyms, abbreviations, and jargon. It is easy to fall into using them without realising. When setting out to do meaningful participation it is therefore important to be aware of language use, make sure we are using clear language and spelling things out. From personal lived experience, I have found, sometimes, professionals and others in 'the room' do not know what something means, but feel they should so they do not question it. Using clear language is of benefit to all.

One Person Representing Everyone

Often people with lived experience are asked to 'be the voice' of lived experience, that is, to represent everyone who has lived experience. Or are a lone voice in a room, which everyone turns to in order to represent all lived experience. It goes without saying that there is an abundance of demographic diversity to humans and experiences, that it cannot be possible that one person can represent everyone. Individuals view the world through their 'worldview' of past experiences (Mead 2019: 51) and therefore may not truly know or feel what it means to experience something someone else has. The important thing here is that this is understood and even recognised.

This leads to Equality, Diversity and Inclusion (EDI) in participation work. Often people who come forward are those listened too and heard and therefore seldom heard voices are not. Engaging with people who come forward only is often seen as easier than going out and seeking wider views. It requires time and effort to seek wider views and experiences within participation, but often this is critical. It can be important to reflect on who is 'in the room' and whether demographics represent local populations. If not, services become developed through heard voices only perhaps leading to seldom heard voices being even less heard.

Our own unconscious bias should also be explored, and whether we are leaning towards those who say what we want to hear. Sometimes participation is about hearing difficult experiences, or what has previously gone unspoken and changing the direction of the work if necessary.

Culture

Is participation embedded into what is done and a part of routine practise, or is it only thought about by a few? Sometimes it can be seen to be the responsibility of one person or worker and not anyone else's. Bjønness et al's. study (2020: 5) on participation and shared decision making in CYP mental health inpatients units, discussed 'a culture of "no decision without participation"'. But this needed a culture shift alongside a focus on routinely involving CYP, training for staff, and being flexible to CYPs needs (Bjønness et al. 2020: 6). Culture cannot be underestimated when doing non tokenistic participation. It may need those additional aspects such as training needs to be considered and implemented to work towards it becoming embedded and the norm. Hearing from those who have participated can be a powerful way to shift people's thinking.

Upon starting in a lived experience role once, someone said to me 'I have never worked with someone with lived experience before', in which I said 'wrong, you work with people with lived experience every day, it is just my job role names it'. I have also had 'how should I talk with [person with lived experience]'. I think it is important to explore fears, worries, and concerns in current culture with the wider team and work through them, in my experience, they often come from a want to get things right.

In services, it is often seen as the responsibility of the person coordinating participation to make everyone aware about it and recruit people to participate, yet often they are not connected to CYP and parents and carers through a clinical role. How do CYP/parents and carers know about participation, is it one person's or everyone's responsibility to share information?

Misplaced Intent

For participation to be meaningful, people with lived experience should be involved with a purpose, not just 'because'. Participation is not about asking people with lived experience to be involved in every single thing without a reason. When asking people to participate, it is important to think about 'why', and what the intent, reason, and purpose behind that is. If the answer is along the lines of, it would be good to have people with lived experience in the room, it is felt as the thing to be done or brings a 'nice' touch, then it is a good time to reflect. If we are asking people to bring experiences, which are often attached to a variety of emotions, it is good to have a clear reason, benefit, action plan or the likes behind it.

In the past I have used the example 'Imagine being asked to talk about your most painful life experiences for 30 minutes to a room of 100 people. What would it take? Next time you ask someone with lived experiences to speak about them, think about this'. Of course it goes without saying, not all experiences are painful or difficult, but it is important to remember that at the heart of participation is people talking about their lived experiences who have lives as detailed and complex as our own. Often people are being asked to talk about really difficult times and share really difficult things. It can take courage, vulnerability, and strength to share lived experiences. Asking 'why?' ensures there is a clear purpose to this.

A Summary

This chapter looks into some of the considerations of meaningful engagement has shown there is a range of components to be considered to help shift away from participation experienced as tokenistic. Evidently, local contexts should also inform these considerations. It has shown that active steps need to be taken to prevent participation being experienced as tokenism. Time, support, resources, wider support, personal thoughts and feelings, assumptions, language, representation, culture, and intent are among these considerations.

Conclusion

This chapter has explored what is behind the word tokenism, evidencing there are many factors captured into one word. Ultimately situating the conceptualism of tokenism as experienced as a feeling. It has discussed aspects that may be useful to consider when developing meaningful participation, offering thoughts and narrative around them.

I would like to thank Elizabeth for her contributions to this chapter.

References

Aoki, Y. (2020). Shared decision making for adults with severe mental illness: A concept analysis. *Japan Journal of Nursing Science.* 17(4). [Online] Available at: https://doi.org/10.1111/jjns.12365 [Accessed 19 November 2022].

Arnstein, S. (1969). A ladder of citizen participation. [Online] Available at: https://www.miguelangelmartinez.net/IMG/pdf/1969_Arnstein_participation_ladder_AJP.pdf [Accessed 20 November 2022].

Barrett, J. (2010). User and carer participation and advocacy. In: Richardson, G., Partridge, I. and Barrett, J. *Child and Adolescent Mental Health Services An Operational Handbook.* 2nd ed. London: The Royal College of Psychiatrists. 78–84.

Bjønness, S., Viksveen, P., Johannessen, J. O. and Storm, M. (2020). User participation and shared decision-making in adolescent mental healthcare: A qualitative study of healthcare profess. *Child and Adolescent Psychiatry and Mental Health.* 14 (2), 1–9. [Online] Available at: https://doi.org/10.1186/s13034-020-0310-3 [Accessed 30 October 2022].

Cambridge Dictionary (2022). Tokenism. [Online] Available at: https://dictionary.cambridge.org/dictionary/english/tokenism [Last accessed 15 June 2022].

Department of Health (2002). Learning from Bristol: The Department of Health's response to the report of the public inquiry into children's heart surgery at the Bristol Royal Infirmary 1984–1995. [Online] Available at: https://assets.publishing.service.gov.uk/government/uploads/system/uploads/attachment_data/file/2733 [Accessed 19 November 2022].

Farrington, C. (2016). Co-designing healthcare systems: Between transformation and tokenism. *Journal of the Royal Society of Medicine.* 109 (10), 368–371.

Fleming, J. (2013). Young people's participation - where next? *Children & Society.* 27, 484–495. [Online] Available at: doi:10.1111/j.1099-0860.2012.00442.x [Accessed 5 November 2022].

Foucault, M. (1988). *Madness and Civilization: A History of Insanity in the Age of Reason.* New York: Vintage Books.

Hahn, D., Hoffmann, A., Felzien, M., LeMaster, J., Xu, J. and Fagnan, L. (2017). Tokenism in patient engagement. *Family Practice*. 34 (3), 290–295.

Hart, R.A. (1992). *Children's Participation: From Tokenism to Citizenship*. Florence: UNICEF, International child development centre.

Hayes, D., Edbrooke-Childs, J., Town, R., Wolpert, M. and Midgley, N. (2018). Barriers and facilitators to shared decision making in child and youth mental health: Clinician perspectives using the Theoretical Domains Framework. *European Child & Adolescent Psychiatry*. 28, 655–666. [Online] Available at: https://doi.org/10.1007/s00787-018-1230-0 [Accessed 20 November 2022].

Hitchen, S., Watkins, M., Williamson, G.R., Ambury, S., Bemrose, G., Cook, D. and Taylor, M. (2011). Lone voices have an emotional content: Focussing on mental health service user and carer involvement. *International Journal of Health Care Quality Assurance*. 24(2).

Law, D., Faulconbridge, J. and Laffan, A. (2015). Appendix 4: Outcome monitoring in children and young people's mental health systems in The Child & Family Clinical Psychology Review. *The British Psychological Society*. 3, 34–36.

Lundy, L. (2018). In defence of tokenism? Children's right to participate in collective decision-making. [Online] Available at: https://pureadmin.qub.ac.uk/ws/portalfiles/portal/148759327/Tokenismfin.pdf [Accessed 20 November 2022].

Macgregor, A. (2022). Meaningful participation or tokenism for individuals on community based compulsory treatment orders? Views and experiences of the mental health tribunal in Scotland. *Journal of Mental Health*. 31(2), 158–165.

Majid, U. (2020). The dimensions of tokenism in patient and family engagement: A concept analysis of the literature. *Journal of Patient Experience*. 7 (6), 1610–1620.

Mead, S. (2019). Narrative practice and intentional peer support: A conversation between Hamilton Kennedy and Sherry Mead. *International Journal of Narrative Therapy and Community Work* (4), 50–55.

Mercer, A., O'Curry, S., Donnan, J., Stedmon, J., Reed, J. and Griggs, H. (2015). Delivering psychological services for children and young people with physical health needs and their families in The Child & Family Clinical Psychology Review. *The British Psychological Society*. 3, 71–83.

Ocloo, J. and Matthews, R. (2016). From tokenism to empowerment: Progressing patient and public involvement in healthcare improvement. *BMJ Quality & Safety*. 25 (8), 626–632.

Pollard, B.J. (1993). Autonomy and paternalism in medicine. *Medical Journal of Australia*. 159 (11–12),797–802.

Strickler, D.C. (2009). Addressing the imbalance of power in a traditional doctor-patient relationship. *Psychiatric Rehabilitation Journal*. 32(4), 316–318. [Online] Available at: doi:10.2975/32.4.2009.316.318 [Accessed 1 November 2022].

The Bristol Royal Infirmary Inquiry (2001). The Report of the Public Inquiry into children's heart surgery at the Bristol Royal Infirmary 1984–1995. [Online] Bristol Inquiry. Available at: http://www.bristol-inquiry.org.uk/final_report/the_report.pdf [Accessed 19 November 2022].

Walker, L. (2020). What do children and young people want and need from nurses (and therapists?). In: Baldwin, L. (Ed). *Nursing Skills for Children and Young People's Mental Health*. Switzerland: Springer. 21–36.

Warming, H. (2011). Children's participation and citizenship in a global age: Empowerment, tokenism or discriminatory disciplining. *Social Work & Society.* 9 (1).

Willig, C. (2019). Ontological and epistemological reflexivity: A core skill for therapists. *Therapists and Knowledge.* 19(3), pp.186–194. [Online] Available at: https://doi.org/10.1002/capr.12204 [Accessed 19 November 2022].

Chapter 4

The Benefits and Challenges of Participation for Children and Young People

Anna Wilson

Introduction

At age 15, sat rather anxiously amongst other CAMHS (Child and Adolescent Mental Health Services) patients for the first time at my local participation group, I would never have believed how life changing my participation journey would be or that it would culminate in compiling a chapter for a book about participation in child and adolescent mental health.

This chapter collates the first-hand accounts of the benefits of participation from young people who have lived experience of accessing mental health services in the UK. Their collective experiences of participation include individual care, local and national NHS participation groups as well as involvement with national charities and research groups. Undoubtably their involvement in participation has played a role in their ability to share their experiences in such a candid and poignant way. The role participation has played in the recovery, growth, and development of these incredible young people shines through in the words written. This chapter is spilt into experiences of participation at an organisational level followed by experiences of individual participation in their own care.

These personal narratives make it clear that the benefits of participation extend beyond service improvement to support recovery and create a safe space where young people feel heard and valued among peers that understand the difficulties of mental illness. Increased confidence and self-esteem were repeatedly mentioned as well as the impact of feeling valued and being able to give something back to the service and other young people. Longer-term benefits include impact of career choice and the development of lifelong friendships.

Although there is a growing evidence base and number of research papers on patient participation at an organisational level in mental health services, there ironically appears to be a lack of research focusing on young people's experiences of participation in their own words, particularly the benefits to them. Most of the research appears to focus on the process of participation, service improvements, acceptability of

DOI: 10.4324/9781003288800-4

participation, professionals' views, and challenges faced. It appears the potentially enormous personal benefits young people experience when being involved in organisational-level participation have largely been overlooked. However, some research has found that when young people are involved in organisation participation it increases their confidence and self-esteem (Allan and Travers-Hill, 2019; Coates and Howe, 2014; Cole, 2019) improves social skills (Coates and Howe, 2014) and they learn other new skills (Dunn and Mellor, 2017).

Background and Reasons for Getting Involved in Organisational-level Participation

A number of young people kindly and openly contributed their experiences to the chapter including their reasons for becoming involved in participation.

> After spending nearly 9 months in an adolescent psychiatric hospital, I moved to a new area which meant that I had to go to a new community CAMHS service. Due to struggling with meeting new people and feeling uncomfortable talking about my feelings and experiences, I found it difficult to begin with to engage with my CAMHS worker and so I was asked if I wanted to be involved in the participation group within the service.
>
> (Sophie)

> I experienced my first serious mental health crisis at 16 as a result of an intense clash of personal factors that suddenly occurred at the time. Because of my age, however, I feel that my experiences of accessing CAMHS were somewhat doomed from the start. By the time I was finally being regularly seen by my local service, I was already fast approaching my 18th birthday, and therefore quickly found myself sucked into the murky haze that lingers between CAMHS and adult services, with no real direction, support or direct referral, despite having only just been prescribed my first mood stabiliser at the height of my A-Levels. Living in a rural area with limited transport only exacerbated my sense of isolation. On finishing school, I was woefully unprepared to move away to university, but attempted to do so anyway, without any support from services, which only initiated a series of further crises for the next few years before I was settled into an adult service much later on.
>
> Generally, aside from one supportive CPN (Community Psychiatric Nurse), my experiences of CAMHS were poor. However, I was never advised on how I could share my feedback, and I was certainly never signposted to a participation group or worker in my local service –

I'm not sure one even existed. Instead, my introduction to participation first came about through regional and national work in the voluntary sector, leading to paid sessional work for other organisations as a young advisor.

(Jude – He/Him)

I'm 25 now but I was 16 when I accessed CAMHS. I was experiencing depression and anxiety after being bullied in school and struggled a lot with social anxiety especially. When I think back, it was such a hard time for me but things began to change during my involvement in CAMHS. I started to access Cognitive Behavioural Therapy (CBT), where I worked with a therapist around what I was experiencing. A key part of my therapy was working on my anxiety to be able to socialise. My therapist explained to me about the participation group the service had and how it was made up of other young people with experience of mental health difficulties. I didn't know it then but it ended up being a key part of my therapy work and working through the social anxiety I was experiencing.

(Amy – She/Her)

My name is Beth, and ever since the beginning of high school I've suffered with mental health issues. I've always wanted to make a change in the way mental health issues are perceived, thus participation became my way to help make a change. Participation is incredibly important to me; it gives me a pathway to express myself and my opinions on mental health and the mental health system, and I feel as though I'm finally speaking out about what so many young people with mental health issues want to say, but don't have the voice nor the platform to!

(Beth)

I started accessing CAMHS when I was 15 due to struggling with anxiety and depression. I was very grateful for the support I received from CAMHS however there were areas of my care that I felt could have been improved. I initially got involved in my local participation group in main because I was asked and at the time tended to always say yes. However, realising that my experience could help improve services led me to seeking out national and research involvement opportunities.

(Anna)

Supporting Recovery

Participation and involvement at an organisational level is not specifically aimed at being therapeutic in nature and is often coordinated by non-clinical staff. Nevertheless, it is clear from these narratives that the effect organisation participation has on supporting recovery should not be underestimated.

> I was sceptical of this at first but I went along and after that, I never stopped going and it played a huge part in my recovery... I eventually felt more comfortable around the people I had met, which encouraged me to engage with my CAMHS worker and work on my journey to recovery.
>
> (Sophie)

> I have no doubt that the opportunities that participation offered me, the inspiring other young people I worked with, our outstanding adult mentors, and all we collectively achieved, equipped me with everything I needed to start to chisel my own path along my journey of recovery after a rocky initial experience of trying to access help. I hope other children and young people are encouraged to have such an opportunity, too.
>
> (Jude – He/Him)

> The jump between services and discharge (inpatient and then outpatient) can be a huge and overwhelming gap. Having the participation group acted as a step between. It helped to make transitions more bearable reducing the chance of relapsing ... Participation work gave me a focus and a reason to keep well, which can be an extremely hard thing to find when struggling with mental illness. The reason why I kept coming back to the group was simple; it acted as the final missing piece in my journey to recovery ... it was where recovery truly began.
>
> (Bella)

> My therapist explained to me about the participation group the service had and how it was made up of other young people with experience of mental health difficulties. I didn't know it then but it ended up being a key part of my therapy work and working through the social anxiety I was experiencing ... Participation firstly, was an important part of my therapy, in being a safe space to test out my thoughts, feelings and behaviour and how they all linked. This was important in helping me work through my mental health struggles and test out different things.
>
> (Amy – She/Her)

> Participation was a non-judgemental place to try and discover who I was again as I had been putting on a façade for so long.
>
> (Amy – She/Her)

Opportunity to Connect with Others Experiencing Mental Illness

Mental illness can be an extremely isolating experience especially so when going through this as a young person; a time of huge change which often comes with a pressure to 'fit in' with peers. Therefore, it is unsurprising the tremendous benefit gained through connecting with other young people going through similar experiences. Being seen and understood is fundamental to positive social interaction, but it can be difficult find, particularly due to the stigma still surrounding mental illness. When reading the experiences below it is heart-warming to see the power of connecting with others through participation and the longevity of friendships gained.

> Being part of the local CAMHS participation group allowed me to connect with other young people with mental illness during a time in my life where I felt incredibly lonely and isolated. It was a safe space for me where I didn't have to put on a brave face or pretend that I was ok. I met two of my closest friends who I still regularly see 10 years on from when I first joined the participation group.
>
> (Anna)

> I was able to meet new people and build lifelong friendships with people who had been through similar experiences that I had and had used CAMHS services themselves.
>
> (Sophie)

> The experience of meeting and collaborating with other young people from up and down the country with similar experiences for the first time was hugely beneficial to me in different ways … I had an invaluable opportunity to meet other young people with similar experiences for the first time, creating opportunities for peer support and building resilience. Having grown up in a rural area with no group opportunities offered to me in my own service, this had a great personal impact on me.
>
> (Jude – He/Him)

> We are all in the same boat, having been where each other has, perhaps in different ways or times but with an understanding that is hard to find in those who have not. The non-judgmental, accepting environment that the group offers, provided me with the opportunity to make new friends and to feel important again.
>
> (Bella)

> These friends were invaluable to me and were the main part of changing my mental health around. We laughed and joked and met every

day over the summer holidays. Even to this day, they are still my most important friends, and we look after each other through thick and thin. The main thing that helped was the fact that they were at CAMHS, for their own particular reason, if anything we were all in the same boat trying to stay afloat. Staying afloat was easy when you have the understanding and acceptance from good friends without any judgemental behaviour .... I was able to build a network of people around me which I have been able to rely on within the last 10 years.

(Amy – She/Her)

Between the ages of 16 and now, we have all remained friends and have been there for each other during the worst and the best times. I see this as an ongoing benefit from participation. One was even the celebrant at my wedding ... As our friendships grew, off shoots came out of the participation space we had created, amazingly we began to socialise outside of the group and outside of the service and engage in 'everyday life' activities together. Before participation, I had social anxiety which had prevented me doing these things. We began meeting weekly at a coffee shop to just chat, laugh and catch up. It felt like participation enabled us to take that step into the real world on our own independently of services.

(Julia – She/Her)

Improving Confidence and Self-esteem

Adolescence is a time that many people struggle with low confidence and low self-esteem. Given that speaking during meetings is something that adults often find difficult it highlights how incredible these young people (many of whom struggled significantly with low self-esteem) are to become involved in participation and speak out about their experiences to drive positive change. As shown below, participation when done correctly can be used as a vessel to increase confidence through showing young people their value and capability.

Participation helped me build my confidence as I was involved in many different projects which required me to speak in front of many people and share my experiences/ideas, which I previously would never have done.

(Sophie)

The professional opportunities and improvement to my overall well-being enabled my confidence to soar. The impact on my overall sense of self-worth and self-esteem was significant and made me feel like I had something unique and important I could contribute to the development of services as well as to other young people.

(Jude – He/Him)

It provided me with the opportunity to build up my confidence and independence back up again.

(Bella)

We learnt about public speaking and speaking confidently in front of other people. Participation gave me social confidence in being myself, making friends gave me the confidence to do things. If I was thrown into a meeting and told to do public speaking, I wouldn't have done it but for me it was the fact that all my friends that I had made in the group were doing it, that I then took part. These are skills I have taken with me into my life and who I am today.

(Amy – She/Her)

My confidence and willingness to speak my thoughts on challenging and sensitive topics has really increased since I started on the panel with young minds; I no longer feel afraid to talk about my darkest times and how I got through them, and I feel such an element of pride for finally being able to do so.

(Beth)

Although a safe space I was often very much outside of my comfort zone, with the support of participation workers and surrounded by people that I trusted I was able to speak in professional meetings and present at conferences. Participation surrounded me by people that believed in me and my abilities during a time that I had no belief in myself. Slowly the confidence that others had in me started to develop into confidence that I had in myself.

(Anna)

Feeling Valued, Heard, and Giving Back to the Service

Being able to be part of improving services through participation, allowed me to give something back to the service which had saved my life … Participation has such a huge therapeutic value for young people, as I believe it makes young people feel like they are a critical part of the service, they are valued, and their voices are heard.

(Sophie)

I was grateful to have some kind of opportunity to share my own experiences and thoughts for the first time, having felt so isolated and unheard during my time as a service user. One thing was certain – I was insistent that I didn't want other young people in my local area to feel the same. These opportunities enabled me to see first-hand how sharing experiences and stories can make a difference, whether it was challenging the perspective of a senior clinician, educating MPs, or helping another young person to find their voice.

After a disheartening, frustrating experience of accessing services myself, becoming involved in participation and seeing how my story and experiences could somehow help others gave my own wellbeing a huge boost, too.

(Jude – He/Him)

Throughout the months of attending the participation group I slowly began to leave the place that for so long had felt like the 'norm' for me. At the same time, I helped other people to do the same. For too long we had each felt like the person needing the help and after so long you begin to resent the reality of that. So knowing you can give back and help another person in your situation takes away some of that frustration.

(Bella)

As part of the Participation group, we created a safe space to express our own feelings on how to improve the service whilst also taking into account other users' recommendations. We made our group known through fundraising, holding various events and working alongside CAMHS to improve the waiting room area with young people and parents. Even though participation was a small fraction of the work being done at CAMHS, it was a major necessity in ensuring all users to the service felt safe, without guilt and most importantly valued.

(Julia)

When I had overcome my mental health struggles, I found that I really wanted to give back and this then led to me taking on a national young advisor participation role, where I was able to use my experiences to influence larger pieces of work.

(Amy – She/Her)

I've always wanted to make a change in the way mental health issues are perceived, thus participation became my way to help make a change. Participation is incredibly important to me; it gives me a pathway to express myself and my opinions on mental health and the mental health system, and I feel as though I'm finally speaking out about what so many young people with mental health issues want to say, but don't have the voice nor the platform to! Participation in mental health services is so, so incredibly important; not only does it help young people be heard, improve their confidence and ability to open up, it also gives the services an insight into the mind of people who have access to such services.

(Beth)

Participation gave me a space where people understood that I was hurting and may need extra support, but that I still had something valuable to contribute to improving mental health care.

(Anna)

Impact on Career

The impact of participation on those involved doesn't end when young people stop attending a participation group. The skills gained and confidence acquired are not lost and continue into the next phase of a person's life, manifesting a tangible impact on future career.

I gained so many new skills through participation and I have been able to continue using these skills and this experience in my future, as I then went on to qualify as a mental health nurse and now work in CAMHS.

(Sophie)

One of the key benefits of participation was how it kickstarted my whole career in mental health and peer support, and how it directly impacted on my professional development. Participation also introduced me to aspects of politics and government work I wasn't aware of, introduced me to important contacts from around the country, and gave me invaluable work experience I simply could not have gained elsewhere. I have since developed a career working in peer support and creating spaces for others to safely share their own experiences based on the inspiration and motivation I experienced in those settings.

(Jude – He/Him)

Being part of a participation group really helped me built up my CV and gave me lots to write about in my university application. Without the experience participation gave me and the confidence instilled in me through having a voice, I doubt that I would have had the confidence to pursue a career in research and medicine.

(Anna)

Supported Skill Development

I did a huge amount of public speaking to a variety of different audiences at conferences and meetings of various sizes, for example, and for a while I also had a unique opportunity to co-chair a CYP IAPT service development group alongside senior clinicians and professionals as a young person. There was also a strong learning curve, however, and a real challenge at times – even learning how to confidently travel and commute independently around the country was a big deal!

(Jude – He/Him)

In the more formal participation meetings we would take on different roles that as young people we wouldn't have normally been able to take on in other spaces such as being treasurer, writing minutes and I even really enjoyed being the Chair of the group and Chairing meetings for a time period. During my time in participation I developed many skills during the work we did together, a key one was social skills and managing my anxiety.

(Amy – She/Her)

As part of the participation group we received formal training on service evaluation, project management, leadership, and communication skills.

(Anna)

Individual Participation

Individual participation refers to patient involvement in shared decision making about care and treatment with their health professionals. Compared to organisational-level participation, there is a greater amount of research in this area that considers the views of young people using mental health services. Sadly, a lot of research into this area suggests that individual participation and shared decision making is not always done well, which is reflected in the narratives shared below.

Research suggests that there is a multitude of barriers to effective individual participation; clinicians expressed concerns that standardised treatment pathways and regulations that had to be followed with no flexibility to deviate based on individual client needs, additionally they reported that they don't have enough time to build a relationship so that young people feel safe (Bjønness et al., 2020). A systematic review into user involvement found that several studies showed that adolescents experienced limited treatment options, lack of involvement in the decision-making process, and lack of opportunities to voice their opinions (Viksveen et al., 2022). These findings very much reflect Ben's personal experience of accessing services:

> Most of the sessions consisted of advice that was very general to someone experiencing the types of issues I was facing. At no point did it feel like the clinician was interested in helping me through my situation. Rather, it felt like they aimed to move me through the process as quickly as possible... At points in the sessions, it felt more like an interview than a dialogue.

Research into individual participation in inpatient units found that young people had "no real involvement in decision making" (Martin, 2019: 176). The use of observations from staff were used as substitutes for and mis-interpretations of what young people where actually feeling or experiencing. Decisions were made based on these staff observations and not through conversation with the actual young person being treated (Martin, 2019). Another study reported that young people required more information and understanding if their care is to enable them to be involved in decision making (Bjønness et al., 2020). At a minimum, young people should understand the rational for the decisions made about their care and how this affects them, it is disheartening to see that this basic foundation of shared decision making is being neglected.

Below, Ben openly shares his personal experiences, which reflect what has been found in research, highlighting the hugely detrimental effects of lack of individual level participation. His experiences particularly show how much can be gained for effective individual participation in care and shared decision making.

Ben Sharp's (He/Him) Story

A key difference between my experience of NHS and private healthcare settings was the extent to which I felt I had a choice in terms of my clinician. When I sought treatment with the NHS it always felt like I was going to be put with someone. I didn't feel as though I had the ability to find the clinician that was right for me as this was never emphasised during the process. When I sought treatment through private healthcare, the idea of choice was always emphasised. At all stages of the process, I understood that if I didn't 'click' with the first clinician I could be paired with a different one. This allowed me to approach the initial sessions in a different way. Rather than my mental healthcare feeling like a slog through assigned sessions, I was able to view the relationship as a partnership. I had a greater level of agency in terms of my mental healthcare.

This increased agency was helpful for a few reasons. Firstly, it allowed me to be more open in my sessions. This was because I was able to have a more even dialogue with my clinician. I was able to be a lot more relaxed in my initial sessions because I knew that it was not the 'be all and end all'. I knew if this clinician wasn't a good fit there would be other options, so there wasn't as much pressure to make it work the first time. Secondly, this increased agency allowed me more opportunity to grow within the sessions. Because it felt like I was choosing to go, I felt more comfortable in sharing things with my clinician. This meant that it was easier to make progress as it was easier to directly approach my issues. My clinician felt like someone I could trust rather than someone I was being forced to see. Finally, this increased agency allowed me to build a positive relationship with my clinician more easily. Because it felt like I was being matched with the right person rather than being put with whoever was available, the relationship felt more even. This meant that sessions felt less intimidating as it felt like the clinician was on my side.

In terms of the content of the sessions, my level of participation as the patient had a great effect on the experience of mental healthcare. My first experience of mental healthcare, which I had when I was younger was a negative experience. I felt like I was being forced to attend therapy with a person who wasn't on my side and was someone I didn't like. My more recent experience was a lot more positive, and a key reason for this positivity was my level of participation.

One of the main reasons for the negativity in my initial experience was the lack of personalisation given in the sessions. The advice I was given in the initial sessions felt very 'off the shelf'. Most of the sessions consisted of advice that was very general to someone experiencing the types of issues I was facing. At no point did it feel like the clinician was interested in helping me through my particular situation. Rather, it felt like they aimed to move me through the process as quickly as possible. This was especially unhelpful to me as a younger patient as it contributed to the element of intimidation already present in opening a dialogue with a previously unknown adult. At points in the sessions, it felt more like an interview than a dialogue. Rather than being afforded the opportunity to work through my issues, I was simply being asked why I hadn't done certain things.

As a neurodiverse patient, I have issues independent of mental health-care in terms of relating to someone I don't know. The lack of my parti-cipation as a patient strengthened these pre-existing issues. Because the sessions were not tailored to me, I was not able to build a strong rela-tionship with my clinician. The generality of most of the content of the sessions meant that the specifics of my situation weren't addressed. While the advice may have worked for someone with similar issues purely in terms of mental health, it was not particularly helpful for a patient, such as me, who has social issues independent of my mental health. If the session had been more tailored to my specific needs, progress would have been more quickly made. The generality of my sessions meant it felt like I was going round in circles as my clinician would, week after week, give me the same advice that didn't work. By allowing me participation in terms of the direction of their care, it would have become far easier for my specific issues to be solved.

The increased element of collaboration between me and my clinician led to a much more positive experience in my more recent care. When entering sessions my needs were always emphasised. At all times I knew that the purpose of the sessions was to help me, rather than to move me through the system. This meant that I was more easily able to address my specific issues. Progress was made much more quickly as I was given targeted help. I had the ability to go in and to work through an issue that was troubling me. There was no longer the repetitiveness present in my prior experience, this meant that we were able to move through issues rather than becoming stuck in the same place each time I entered a session.

Another thing this increased participation offered me was the opportunity to build a much stronger partnership with my clinician. Because I had a greater level of participation, I was able to build a relationship with my clinician before starting to address my issues. As someone who had found the general idea of mental healthcare intimidating, this was extremely helpful. I was able to create a strong bedrock to build on top of, which meant that the following sessions were more effective. The increased level of participation meant that I was able to find a form of mental healthcare that really suited me. The sessions were able to be more guided by my needs as a patient rather than being completely guided by the clinician.

Final Thoughts/Conclusion

I sincerely hope that reading the positive effect both individual and organisational participation has had on these young people has helped to inspire and ignite a passion to make participation an essential part of mental health services. Service users have so much to gain from being involved in participation, but also so much to give to improve services.

To conclude this chapter on benefits of participation from the perspective of young service users, here are some final views that I felt really highlight just how valuable, and life-changing participation can be:

> Personally, my own mental health made me feel extremely alone and without a voice. Participation changed all that and made me feel empowered, confident and with a voice that is appreciated. This helped me going forward with my life.

Looking back, participation was a solid foundation in which to grow from and continue moving forward with my life. I have a core group of friends who will continue to be there for me and me there for them, the impact of this cannot be underestimate.

Participation has certainly moulded me into the stronger person I am today.

If you take anything away from this chapter, make it that personalised care is of upmost importance.

Participation work provided me with a great transition back into the world of work and a return to routine, and made me realise that I could work and have a job, as when I was younger I was worried that might not be possible given my health needs.

References

Allan, S. M. and Travers-Hill, E. (2019). "Service user interview panels for recruitment to UK Child and Adolescent Mental Health Services: A questionnaire study exploring the experiences of young people, staff and candidates", *Patient Experience Journal*, 6(3), pp. 50–54. Available at: https://doi.org/10.35680/2372-0247.1360.

Bjønness, S. *et al.* (2020). "User participation and shared decision-making in Adolescent Mental Healthcare: A qualitative study of healthcare professionals' perspectives", *Child and Adolescent Psychiatry and Mental Health*, 14(1). Available at: https://doi.org/10.1186/s13034-020-0310-3.

Coates, D. and Howe, D. (2014). "The importance and benefits of youth participation in mental health settings from the perspective of the headspace Gosford Youth Alliance in Australia", *Children and Youth Services Review*, 46, pp. 294–299. Available at: https://doi.org/10.1016/j.childyouth.2014.09.012.

Cole, L. (2019). *Young People's Narrative Accounts of Participation in the Design and Delivery of NHS Mental Health Services*. Thesis.

Dunn, V. J. and Mellor, T. (2017). "Creative, participatory projects with Young People: Reflections over Five Years", *Research for All*, 1(2), pp. 284–299. Available at: https://doi.org/10.18546/rfa.01.2.05.

Martin, K. (2019). *A Critical Realist Study of Shared Decision-making in Young People's Mental Health Inpatient Units*. Thesis.

Viksveen, P. *et al.* (2022). "User involvement in adolescents' mental healthcare: A systematic review", *European Child & Adolescent Psychiatry*, 31(11), pp. 1765–1788. Available at: https://doi.org/10.1007/s00787-021-01818-2.

Chapter 5

The Benefits and Challenges of Participation for Children and Young People's Mental Health Services and Those Working Within Them

Sarah Gray (She/Her)

Introduction

Having worked in Children's Mental Health Services, Social Care, the Third, and independent sectors for over 40 years I have witnessed a gradual rise in participation and the direct involvement of young people and carers in the services they receive. I have been an advocate of participation since working with a group of care leavers in Nottingham in 1987. The young people, a few colleagues, and I organised and ran a conference about leaving care at which all of the workshops and keynote speeches were co-facilitated by a young person with care experience. The response from conference delegates was very positive and we hoped to include young peoples' lived experience in future service design within the care setting. However, the response from the senior managers and commissioners of services for Children in Care was less enthusiastic and sadly the efforts of those young people, whilst applauded at the time, were not instrumental in changing the status quo. However, that was 35 years ago, and things have moved on. Since then, I have continued to recognise and promote the value of young people and carers taking a role in the development of services that affect them.

I joined South Derbyshire Child and Adolescent Mental Health Services (CAMHS) in August 2004 and am now the Clinical Lead of the Service. I am proud to have worked alongside many colleagues, young people, and carers who actively promote participation and ensure that the service develops with lived experience at its core. South Derbyshire CAMHS now employs both young people and carers, and a Participation Team has developed offering support to young people and carers alike as well as consulting with stakeholders, managers, commissioners, and clinicians. The team are involved in interviews, facilitating support groups, running a telephone helpline, service development meetings, and are regularly called upon by the wider NHS Trust and our local commissioners

DOI: 10.4324/9781003288800-5

to advise on specific projects. In past years, we have been successful in becoming a trailblazer site in the Young Minds 'Amplified' project to help promote participation within the service, and more recently successfully applied for funding from the Charlie Waller Trust for a permanent parent/carer role to join and work alongside our young person Expert by Experience.

When speaking to colleagues today who work in Children and Young People's Menth Health services (CYPMHS), there is an almost unanimous response that participation is a good thing, it is helpful, and we must have more. But what does that actually mean in reality? Do people really understand the benefits at a personal, systemic, and community level? Have people challenged their own preconceived and somewhat prejudiced ideas about letting go of power, losing their jobs to the "unregistered", and fully embracing a new addition to the workforce at every level?

In this chapter I hope to explore some of those benefits and challenges of participation for CYPMHS and those working within them with the help of professionals, young people, parents, and carers from across the country. In the true spirit of participation, in order to gather views I circulated an anonymous and confidential survey, sharing across networks to seek responses from a broad range of people, and collated the results (See Appendix 1 at the end of the chapter for questions). Some responses surprised me but, overall, I was impressed with the honesty of respondents. The information from that survey, as well as my first-hand experience, has formed the basis of this chapter. I have also been able to take some information and apply it to the CAMHS in which I work. I hope that as well as being informative, other services looking to implement participation can learn from this chapter and take aspects into their own services also.

The survey responses received came from the following groups: young people both involved in participation and not, commissioners from Clinical Commissioning Groups who ultimately make decisions about how funding is allocated, teachers, local authority consultant for education, principal psychologists working with children and young people, clinical leads from CAMHS, parents with lived experience of a child accessing CAMHS, service managers of CAMHS, clinical staff working in CYPMH, carers of children with experience of care, social care staff, and people with no experience of CYPMHS at all. I hoped to reach a broad range of people with the questionnaire in order to consider how participation affects and impacts people from many different perspectives. I received over 50 responses from across the country.

I hope that people who read this chapter can see how participation in young people's mental health can have a positive effect on the individual, systems, clinicians, and strategic development of services. I hope that people who have been wondering about getting involved in participation will take the plunge, despite the challenges and there are quite a few, which will be discussed later on in the chapter. Ultimately, I believe that the accounts from young people, parents or carers, and staff within CYPMHS speak for themselves and I hope to demonstrate that participation itself can improve outcomes for young people with mental health difficulties, reduce length of stay in services, provide better value for money, improve accessibility for all parts of the community, improve job satisfaction for staff, and improve public perception of CAMHS.

Pros and Cons of Data Collection

The survey was sent out nationwide via a network of colleagues, parents, carers, professionals, and young people. Over 50 responses were received, many of whom are already involved in participation in some form. However, many others felt alienated and excluded from the services that they receive and were keen to see an increase in sustainable models of participation. Due to the anonymous nature of the survey, I was not able to ensure that the responses were coming from all the different groups of people that I wanted to reach. I was not able to confirm that the survey responses came from a culturally diverse, inclusive, and differently abled group of people.

The confidential nature of the survey enabled people to respond honestly and raise concerns as well as compliments about their local services. This also meant that those services could not be identified and so a clear national picture was not available.

For ease and brevity, when speaking about children and young people, I will use the words "young people". I will also use the word "carers" when speaking about parents and carers. The term participation and co-production are used interchangeably to cover involvement in a young person's own care as well as service development and support to others via peer support delivered by both young people and carers.

As the survey was confidential, responders will be only identified as 'young person 1', 'carer 4' etc. Unless specifically stated, as the survey was circulated nationwide (England) responses do not relate to a specific CYPMHS or locality.

Young People

In this section, responses from young people will be discussed. The overall unanimous message was that young people were all in favour of participation and co-production of services. It was highlighted that involvement in participation had a positive impact on a person's self-esteem, overall mental health, and helped young people move from a position of receiving a service to feeling as though they were helping others and being listened to.

Young person 3 said

> Being able to give young people a voice within services that support them will always be an improvement. So many young people feel invalidated and as if their thoughts and ideas don't matter. In providing that space for them to give their opinions on the current state of CAMHS and provide ideas [on] how to improve it and actually be listened to is something that is so crucial to CAMHS and pretty much any service.

Young person 3 also wrote

> My own mental health definitely improved. Being part of a group dedicated to listening to young people's voices and improving the service made me realise that people genuinely care, and it was so nice to be part of a group with those beliefs of making sure young people's voices are heard.

The suggestion here is that, by just ensuring that a forum is available and accessible for young people, a different view of the world is offered, challenging the notion that adults are not interested in what they have to say, and this can help young people to feel validated and cared for. However, young people are also quick to point out that funding, cultural shifts, and a willingness from senior management all remain challenges to participation and still present significant obstacles.

Young person 8 pointed out: "Cultural shifts are slow, and participation has not been a priority before or has been done in a tokenistic way."

Young people frequently reported some experience of participation being tokenistic, that it stopped at certain managerial levels, they were not invited to some meetings, and did not receive enough feedback about suggestions that were given. The youth work toolbox identifies that "A significant part of managing expectations is continually providing feedback throughout the process... If you don't feedback, young people will assume that you don't take any notice of what they have said and lose confidence in your service" (Brown 2014: 54).

Missed opportunities was a theme from several young people and young person 3 added "There are more [future] opportunities to have the voice of young people and families at higher levels of decision making and service design." This suggests that young people perceive participation happening at a certain level and then it stops, or perhaps they receive no feedback when their ideas are acted upon or discussed in other meetings.

Young person 3 shared that their experience having been in a mental health crisis meant that they were even more excluded from decision making, both about their own care and also service development.

> I feel I was not being listened to, simply because I was in such an intense mental health crisis. I still wanted to be listened to. Just because I was in crisis doesn't mean my suggestions on improving the service are invalid. And I think it may have even helped me not feel so useless and such.

This is an extremely important point that was made several times. Just the experience of being involved in participation, being taken seriously, and being listened to, had, and can have, a positive impact on the mental health of those young people and their families. It is also a challenge to services; how do we involve young people in crisis in a safe and respectful way that validates their experience and feelings?

Another important point made was to ensure that when young people are invited to attend meetings or to give suggestions that they are supported in doing so. Many young people reported that their confidence grew because of being part of meetings, being listened to and taken seriously. It was through these experiences that they became able to challenge clinicians, managers, and commissioners and true participation was felt to be in place. However, it is important to note that the power imbalance between a young person and the professionals around the table, if not acknowledged and managed carefully, can be a block to young people and carers speaking out. Thought needs to be given to how that support takes place. For example, it may need to be in place before and after a meeting, by arranging a pre-meeting and a debrief, as well as support during a meeting.

Young person 24 who was employed by a CAMHS identified a challenge that, "The staff are not referring young people to participation and as a lone worker, the challenge of implementing participation across all of the CAMHS teams is a big challenge." This was from a CAMHS with a well-defined participation role. Another cautionary note, that for participation to be truly effective, every part of the system needs to be involved. Several participation workers raised the point that staff are not encouraging young people to attend participation groups and they can sometimes "enter and leave the service without knowing this is an opportunity for them" (young person 24).

Within my own service I am aware that this does happen, clinicians will often cite being too busy, too overwhelmed, and/or too focused on risk to think about referring young people to a participation group. The truth is, however, that by becoming involved in participation young people may move towards independence from services, thus freeing up staff, releasing time for other things and often acting as a mitigation for risks that are present. Education and training, newsletters, and participation staff being present in team meetings can all help to spread the word and encourage staff to help young people attend participation groups or activities.

Young people are clearly telling us that their involvement in participation has a positive impact on their mental health, is likely to mean a shorter time in service and an improvement of overall delivery in CYPMHS. They show incredible insight into their own experience as well as those that have gone before and those to follow. Helping young people to develop those qualities of empathy, compassion and reflective thinking is surely the aim of all services tasked with supporting young people's mental health.

I shall now look at responses from parents and carers.

Parents and Carers

> I truly feel it is a privilege to be part of this work, and have seen (and felt) for myself, that shared understanding, connected, empowered and well supported parent/carers are more resilient, resourceful and better equipped to support their YP's [young people] recovery or ongoing care, and undoubtedly keep the time they spend or rely on clinical services to a minimum.
>
> Carer 14

Carers who responded all supported participation and felt that it should be increased. Carer 18 said, "It has improved our personal experience. It has been helpful listening to others and being given strategies to use … Knowing I can log onto a meeting is reassuring and knowing there is no judgement has been so helpful." This feeling of 'no judgement' is crucial and has been raised several times by carers. It is helpful for services to consider that participation and peer support operate on a premise of 'no judgement' and how helpful this can be for parents often feeling guilt, responsibility, or shame at their young person's mental health difficulties. This is also a useful question for general CYPMHS. Why are carers feeling blamed when their child comes to our services? When the struggle to ask for help and then to access services is hard enough already, this is a good example of how feedback can inform services about how they introduce families to interventions on offer and the language used when talking with families generally.

Many carers commented that if they had received support from another carer whilst waiting for services, they would have been able to manage better and would not need to use other 'crisis' services such as CAMHS duty and Children's Accident and Emergency Departments. In itself, this is an argument for more carer support and efficient use of spending. If we can steer young people away from acute hospital services to more tailor-made interventions, the impact is likely to be positive for young people, carers, and services. Carers also wanted services to be brave enough to listen to the bad experiences and complaints that a service receives. Carer 14 from Derbyshire suggested that CAMHS could "contact families who have historically raised concerns and complaints about CAMHS as a means of giving these families a voice", an opportunity to translate their experiences to positively benefitting future service users. This suggestion was warmly received and supported by the senior leadership team, rein-forcing their commitment for the service to be an open, informed, and co-designed environment based on continuous improvement and best practice.

An overwhelming theme that came from carers' responses was to ensure that families that follow them in accessing services had a better experience then they did, to constantly improve the service, and to use their own experiences to help others. Carer 18 highlighted that giving a voice to those involved will "allow the service to know what are emerging topics / support that is needed for Children and Young People and carers". So, a service informed and led by carers and service users will be responsive and able to adapt to changing mental health challenges for young people.

I am very aware that asking a carer to give up time to be involved in participation activities such as to attend meetings, interviews, training etc. is often unrealistic as in my experience, these activities usually take place Monday–Friday 9am–5pm. Imagine being told that the only way you can contribute to a service that is very dear to your heart is by taking time out of your working day? How would your employer react if this became a regular request? If we are serious and committed to enabling carer invol-vement within CYPMH, then opportunities for full-time employment, paid at an appropriate wage, need to be offered in order for people to change career if that is what they choose to do. Alternatively, such activ-ities should be facilitated with this in mind and perhaps shift culture so meetings where participation input is required happen outside of core business hours. There is one thing for sure, the survey responses indicate carers want to be involved in services, which suggests flexibility to allow this to be important.

Carers also highlighted the lack of involvement in their child's care. Whilst some could see that participation was increasing across some ser-vices, there remains a challenge in appropriate feedback for the people caring for the young person on a daily basis. Carer 5 commented, "Ask parents for feedback. If you give them a chance to say how they think things are going in their child's care, it will improve their confidence and increase their ability to parent and help you do things better." Carer 27 said, "giving feedback will always be better than giving a complaint". If there are options for carers to feedback and this is listened to, taken seriously, and acted upon there may be less need for formal complaints. Carers also noted that offering them a service completely separate to their child's was of little value. This was something that was supported by research conducted in Canada examining caregiver views of youth services (Hawke et al. 2021). Hawke research found that caregivers should be involved in decisions regarding the care the young person received or should be directly involved in the counselling themselves. Participants in Hawke's research also felt that caregivers and young people should be involved in decision-making about service development.

Several parents responding to my questionnaire said that they had a very bad experience with CAMHS, from referral through to discharge. Most located the problems with a lack of communication and felt that increased participation in the services in their area would have been a significant help. Parents understood the pressures on services, but highlighted that this was not an excuse for lack of carer involvement. Parents also highlighted that participation could spotlight great practice. Carer 29 said, "Feedback informs CAMHS where parts of the service are weak and need improvement but equally informs where they are doing well and should be emulated."

Carers were clear that participation needed to be much more embedded in services, even where participation already exists there was a sense there is work to be done.

Carer 14 said,

This is definitely a strategic decision for all stakeholders, and it is impossible to maintain the same level of participation across the entire service. My aspiration would be to develop a team of participation (including peer support) workers across the service and train them to become more actively involved not only supporting families, but clinical staff too, embedded within teams, working with the voluntary sector, in wider community settings, perhaps involved in the delivery of training such as NVR [Non-Violent Resistance training] and treatments, psychoeducation sessions as well as peer support. Real life anecdotal evidence as well as the factual stuff can bring sessions to life and really inspire hope that things can and will get better with the right support. Giving that belief at the right moment is so inspiring and empowering for families.

Carer 14, when asked if they had seen benefits of participation, highlighted a first-hand account from a colleague,

YES!!!!!! Through a work colleague I met many years ago who had received CAMHS support as a teenager and had been involved with an early CAMHS Participation group. She always recounted how this

opportunity literally changed her life – she forged lifelong friendships – her 'go to' in times of celebration or difficulty, as well as
developing an interest and focus in telling her 'story'. It helped her
overcome her own mental health challenges, enhanced her recovery,
and eventually led to her whole career to date being dedicated to
Participation and championing the voice of lived experience.

Carers identified participation as helpful on several levels. They identified
carer fatigue, a sense of blame and guilt as significant barriers for the
recovery of their children. Support from other carers was a way of giving
people hope and enabled them to access strategies and ideas in a non-
judgemental way from people with lived experience alongside the help
they were receiving from services. Carers felt that they and their children
were best placed to help CYPMHS develop co-produced, person-centred,
family focused interventions to ensure.

I will now focus on feedback from clinicians working in CYPMHS.

Clinicians

Clinician feedback on participation highlighted the gaps in knowledge
and information shared with them by management. They were unclear as
to what they could ask the participation staff to become involved in and
they had concerns that participation was service led and not young-
person led. The issue of confidentiality was also raised. Clinician 10 said,
"Unsure about how confidentiality would be upheld if attending all
meetings." Others were clear that this and other issues had to be addressed by offering good training delivered by the participation team to
inform staff of the service and the role of the team. It was felt that these
and other concerns needed to be aired, "name the elephant in the room",
said clinician 17. They suggested that participation staff needed to be
embraced and embedded into the service as colleagues who were subject
to the guidance and with a duty to ensure confidentiality around information governance like any other NHS or public health employee. Within
my own service, the participation team now have access to the electronic
patient records and are treated as any other member of staff. They have
undergone training on information governance, receive clinical, group,
safeguarding and operational supervision, and have an excellent understanding of confidentiality and boundaries. Participation team members
not employed should also have the same opportunity of access to training, ensuring that they felt fully informed and confident in decision
making. Whether they are paid or not for attending this training is a
question for each organisation to decide along with the participation
staff.

Clinicians also highlighted how participation had improved their own practice. Clinician 10 shared, "My own practice has been helped by Participation – I am now more cautious about how collaborative my [1–1] sessions are and recognising the young person's experience."

Clinicians commented that they were incredibly busy, and this sometimes meant that they ran out of time to speak to a young person about participation or referring a carer for peer support. This perhaps highlights that participation can be seen as an additional, rather than an embedded part of the service or routine practice. Others commented that the service needed to equip clinicians with both the time and information to be promoting participation with the young people and carers they work with. Helping staff to see that participation can achieve things such as boosting the confidence of young people and carers alike and then having knock-on benefits such as reducing the time young people need to be receiving a service.

Clinician 11 highlighted that participation can have a positive impact on the morale of staff in CYPMH services, "I would also add that participation maintains connection with those we are working with and the aims of the service when morale is low."

Clinicians were in favour of participation and could recognise its value, although there is clearly still work to be done to ensure that participation staff are embraced as part of the workforce and an understanding that they work to the same standards as others.

The next section looks at feedback received from commissioners working across the field of CYPMH, social care and education.

Commissioners

The response from commissioners was very positive and they were able to take more of a strategic view across all Children's Health Services. Commissioner 2 said,

> I think CAMHS in Derbyshire are very strong regarding participation, in fact I would call it co-production as its better than participation and I also see continuous improvement on this topic. I see CAMHS committing to it in their discussions and actions and by employing experts by experience (EbE), the support they give to them and the real involvement by the EbE. CAMHS staff are fully committed to ensuring they have conversations with CYP [Children and Young People] and their parents regarding plans from the very start and involve them throughout. CAMHS are one of the best examples I have seen re involvement. Excellent work. I see open days, more communication, more understanding of why Participation is important across the system.

The overall sense was that if commissioners are linked in with the participation team they are speaking to the right people and can make decisions and develop services. Commissioner 2 said, "Services are there to meet the needs of the service users – why would you not ask them if you are getting it right?"

A commissioner from a different area pointed out work yet to be done saying,

> I still think it is viewed as an optional extra rather than an essential and is not appropriately funded or given consideration by many senior managers. It also needs to be in place for commissioning not just service delivery. Parents and carers are also not fully included and asked to participate, and this misses out the chance to hear about how services could be improved by the people the CYP [children and young people] live with and who need to support the CYP practically e.g., bring to appointments and to enable them to benefit from the treatment.

All commissioners who replied identified the positives to services, communities, and individuals.

The last section is feedback from managers across CYPMHS.

Managers

One manager raised the issue of diversity amongst participation teams and the importance of ensuring that we have a wide range of voices involved to reflect the communities we serve as well as the diverse experience of young people and their carers. There was also some concern expressed that carer participation could overshadow young people's voices. Manager 6 said, "I think we need a bigger variety of people and a stronger focus on YP Participation." I think this is a valid point, we need to ensure that it is not just the middle-class, white, British voices that are heard, which is often the case. In order to attract more diversity of experience I would suggest that participation teams need to actively go out into communities. We need to acknowledge that our services can be very alienating and frightening for some communities. Creative ways of making mental health services more accessible is a constant challenge, in my own service we run an annual open day where we collaborate with different communities that we serve to attempt to open up and demystify CYPMHS.

Another manager (23) raised the issue of payment for young people and carers' time, "I think representation across all levels of the service, but I think this should be compensated appropriately. Sometimes there is an ask for [young person's] and carer/parent time without payment which is a big ask for time."

Managers highlighted that change often came about after listening to the voice of young people. Manager 41 said,

> Hearing from young people about their experience of coming to CAMHS makes a huge difference. Hearing their voice is more powerful and they notice and see things that practitioners and managers don't notice or see. Young people and carers speaking to senior managers, boards of trust and sharing lived experience appears to be one of the most significant agents for change.

The managers raise some helpful points about diversity and inclusion as well as highlighting that the powerful stories of young people and carers can often be the most helpful and effective when speaking to our organisations about the need for change.

Diversity and Ensuring Access to Participation for All

The issue of inclusion and diversity of experience came up time and time again as a challenge within participation work. "How do we ensure that young people and carers from different ethnic backgrounds feel empowered to get involved?" "LGBTQ+ young people have made a significant impact on participation groups across the country, how do we ensure they remain listened to?" "Young people with a disability are seldom listened to; are they being left out of Participation as well?"

These comments and others made me seriously consider how our own participation team in Derby is predominantly focused on the needs of the service and the issue of inclusion and diversity is rarely discussed. The team and participation groups are encouraged to attend meetings to discuss and review plans for services that have already been planned and commissioned.

An annual World Mental Health Open Day run by Derbyshire CAMHS has provided young people and carers with an opportunity to showcase their work and the work of the wider CAMHS team. This has also had the effect of improving accessibility to the service for all parts of the community as the focus of the day is to challenge the stigma attached to mental health and throw the doors open to the communities in Derby and South Derbyshire. The Open Day is planned and run by the participation team with some help from staff. As carer 3 said "Working on world mental health day was great for the young people it gave them something to focus on and also got their voices heard." The open day also helped to improve job satisfaction for staff who became fully involved as well as improving public and third sector perceptions of the CAMHS.

Personal Views

As I mentioned at the beginning of this chapter my interest and involvement with participation goes back 35 years. I have witnessed first-hand how young people involved in planning, fundraising for, delivering, and reviewing a conference grew in confidence, developed lasting relationships and had an experience where they felt adults took them seriously and trusted them. For young people who had been living in the care system, hurt, and abused within their own families, often excluded from school and work, this was a unique experience and one they expressed they would not forget. Since that time as a Social Worker, Play Therapist, Eating Disorder Specialist and Systemic Family Practitioner, I have tried to ensure that my sessions with young people and family/carers are collaborative. My experience of working therapeutically is that progress is always quicker and more likely to be sustained when a young person feels that they have some control over their own recovery. I know from my own experience that feeling listened to and having your experiences validated as well as your suggestions acted upon can improve your sense of independence, autonomy, and personal achievement and move away from a position of dependence.

My own view of co-production and participation in CYPMH is that it repositions the young person and carers from that of passive service receiver to that of expert of not only their own care, but the service as a whole. It is a challenge and transformation of power and control and can be threatening to those who do not fully understand its benefit. Needham and Carr 2009 in Realpe and Wallace, 2010: 8 highlighted that co-production challenges the notion that service users are passive recipients of a service and are invaluable in helping service development. They went on to say that co-production also requires the involvement of front-line staff to be truly effective (Needham and Carr 2009, in Realpe and Wallace, 2010: 10).

If attempts at participation are ignored or belittled the impact can be devastating, "Co-production with service-users implies a change in everyday routines and relationships of power, and can be met with hostility or withdrawal, which can deepen the crisis of connection in mental health care" (Groot et al. 2022: 238).

I have worked with some truly inspirational young people and carers involved in participation in CAMHS and the transformation I have witnessed is incredible. Their confidence, determination, passion, knowledge and skill has increased exponentially. I have seen young people stand in front of conference audiences and speak, talk to groups of professionals, commissioners and the Boards of NHS Trusts. In fact, the most immediate and sustained change to services has come following these powerful and influential events.

In Derbyshire CAMHS the success and involvement of the participation team in service development cannot be underestimated and has developed over time, but we still have a long way to go.

Challenges and Benefits Identified from the Feedback

The following challenges and benefits have been collated from the responses I received from the questionnaire but also from my own experience over the years and conversations with colleagues, cares, young people and other professionals.

Challenges

1   Participation can be tokenistic if not properly embedded.
2   How you feedback to young people and carers after suggestions have been sought is an extremely important part of the loop and if not done properly can breed mistrust.
3   Managerial structure can sometimes block participation.
4   Ensure appropriate support for young people in attending meetings and making challenges as their confidence grows. This may mean meeting with young people and carers before a meeting to go over the agenda and explain the process as well as support after the meeting has ended.
5   Jargon! Don't use it, or if you do explain what it means.
6   Often participation workers are isolated without the support of a team, think about where they sit, including supervision structures.
7   Participation should not just be at a service level but should include individual care and safety planning to involve carers when appropriate.
8   Don't assume that staff know what participation is and what can be achieved.
9   Be wary that the voice of the parent does not overshadow that of the child or young person.
10 Consideration needs to be given about the power imbalance that some young people, communities and carers experience when accessing mental health services. Try not to replicate this by giving a bigger voice to parents over young people.
11 Try to ensure inclusion in participation and service design for all groups of young people and to develop creative ways of integrating the voices of previously excluded and silenced individuals. Venture out into communities, throw open your doors and invite communities in.
12 Services need to ensure appropriate payment and career development opportunities are available for all involved. Access to training and apprenticeships should be available.

13 Challenge previously held views about confidentiality and ensure that record keeping reflects consent and capacity when it comes to being involved in participation.
14 Funding is always going to be a challenge, diverting money from core CAMHS services is a courageous thing for managers to do but is often essential when starting out in order to demonstrate the impact participation can have on the service delivery.
15 A significant challenge is how do we include young people who are in crisis, clearly their safety and recovery are paramount but maybe consider how participation can be a part of that recovery.

Benefits

1   Just being part of a group can give young people a different perspective, that people care enough to take time to listen to their views and their voice is valued.
2   Being really listened to can positively impact on a young person's mental health and can change their world view to accept that some adults really do care and will listen.
3   Building the confidence of young people increases the likelihood of receiving effective, collaborative challenge thus providing a co-produced direction for service improvement.
4   Improving a carers knowledge of their child's care as well as how the service works and what other support is available can only improve a carers confidence and ability to support their young person in the future.
5   Sharing participation news with staff team can greatly enhance every aspect of the service and is relatively easy to do via newsletter, all staff emails, podcast, webinar, training, attendance at team meetings, etc.
6   A regular review of diversity across the participation community will encourage young people and carers from all backgrounds to become involved in participation.
7   Involvement in participation and the associated benefits can bring a reduction in length of stay in service.
8   Service user satisfaction can increase if people feel they are being listened to, thus a reduction in complaints can follow.
9   A real understanding about the changing and emerging needs of the population can be achieved thus ensuring the best use of scarce resources.
10 Improved morale of staff, across the whole of CYPMHS. Clinicians said that being involved in participation increases their job satisfaction and after all they are there to listen to and help young people. A healthy participation culture tells staff that peoples voices matter, including their own. This can lead to improved staff retention.

11   Commissioning can take place within a collaborative context ensuring that the best of use resources is identified at the point of purchase.
12   Already established networks of young people exist and may be ready, willing and able to offer support to developing services – Young Minds, Anna Freud, Charlie Waller, The Place Network and local CYP IAPT collaboratives and many more.
13   Young people and carers speaking to senior managers and commissioners is the most effective way to bring about change according to the feedback received.
14   Young people and parent/carers develop skills and experience, which can be used on a CV to support any future work applications.
15   Be creative in your thinking and delivery. In Mental Health services we rely heavily on written business plans, data to show improvement and statistics to demonstrate change and value for money. Some of the best presentations I have seen are young people, carers and professionals using more creative ways of getting their message across. Poetry, music, cartoons, artwork, singing and drama are all powerful ways to engage with our communities.

Summary and Recommendations

The overwhelming message from people involved in CYPMHS and those on the periphery is that participation is essential to help services develop to meet the ever-changing needs of the young people and carers we serve. It is clear that there are challenges and that a cultural shift is required across the whole system before real change can be achieved. The positive impact on young people's mental health, self-esteem, confidence and overall ability to reach their potential came up consistently. Whilst no one was saying that CYPMHS are not required the overwhelming feedback was that every aspect of the service would be improved with participation involvement.

The suggestion from the young people that involvement in participation can have a positive impact on their mental health raises the possibility that participation is an intervention in its own right and has a positive impact before any service development work has even begun. A cultural shift in thinking is required for this to be accepted and for participation to be offered routinely as apart of someone's care.

Attention needs to be given to more creative and assertive ways to harness participation from previously excluded groups of young people and carers. We need to look at the diversity of our participation representatives and ensure we are not just consulting with able-bodied, articulate, white, British, heterosexual, middle-class people. If done correctly participation attacks prejudice and power imbalance at every level.

Data still needs to be gathered to ensure that robust evidence shows that participation improves outcomes for young people with mental health difficulties, but anecdotally the connection is clear.

Within my own service, pre-pandemic, the use of Routine Outcome Measures (ROMs) was associated with a reduction in the length of stay in services therefore providing better value for money. The introduction of participation groups to offer a step-down group for young people who no longer require CYPMHS input is an excellent way of ensuring safe discharge and proved to be extremely popular. This also ensured that young people could be rereferred quickly back into the service if the need arose.

Carers reported that they would much prefer to access a service geared towards supporting their young person's mental health rather than using accident and emergency services. Carer support at the point of referral and whilst waiting was highlighted as being a way of avoiding visits to A&E unless necessary and was also a helpful way of being signposted to other services in the meantime.

In conclusion, participation is happening, it is coming to all organisations that provide interventions, health services, education, support etc. to young people. It is not a luxury or an added extra 'when we have the time' but will shape all services in the future and ensure that the limited resources we have are used in the most effective way.

I have never known participation to be unhelpful, challenging and uncomfortable yes, but never unhelpful. Young people's and carers' voices should and must be heard, because once you hear them you won't forget.

Good luck

Appendix I

Participation in CAMHS

1 What is your experience of Participation in Child and adolescent mental health services e.g., Direct involvement, seen it at work, heard about it, etc.?

2 What has been your role in CAMHS e.g., Clinician, Parent, Young Person, Administrator, Manager, Consultant, 3rd Sector, Commissioner, Other professional etc.?

3 Can you give an example of how participation or co-production, in your opinion, has improved CAMHS?

4 What do you see as the challenges and difficulties of implementing participation across CAMHS?

5 Are there areas of the service that you feel would benefit from participation involvement?

6 In your opinion, what level of involvement should the participation team have in CAMHS e.g., no involvement, run support groups,

attend some meetings, attend all meetings, be involved in every level of the service etc?

7 Have you seen any benefits to a young person's mental health from being involved in Participation, e.g., your own, your Child's, a young person you are working with, a young person attending a meeting you have been at, a young person involved in a project at CAMHS etc?

8 Can you think of any reasons why participation should not be part of service improvement in CAMHS?

9 How can participation improve service quality e.g., feedback, voice of the young person, parent involvement etc.?

10 Have you had experience of participation in any other area of health or social care provision and if so, do you have any comments about it?

11 Do you have any other comments about participation and its role in CAMHS?

References

Brown, T. (2014). *Consulting Young People Effectively: A Step-by-Step Guide for Successfully Involving Young People in Decision Making Opportunities.* By Tony Brown of Youth Work Toolbox.

Groot, B., Haveman, A., and Abma, T. (2022). Relational, ethically sound co-production in mental health care research: epistemic injustice and the need for an ethics of care, *Critical Public Health*, 32(2), 230–240, doi:10.1080/09581596.2020.1770694.

Hawke, L. D., Thabane, L., Wilkins, L., Mathias, S., Iyer, S. and Henderson, J. (2021). Don't forget the caregivers! A discrete choice experiment examining caregiver views of integrated youth services. *The Patient*. 14(6), 791–802. [Online]. Available at: doi:10.1007/s40271–40021–00510–00516 [Accessed 24 October 2022].

Realpe, A. and Wallace, L. M. (2010). *What is Co-production?* on behalf of the Coventry University Co-creating Health Evaluation Team. The Health Foundation: London.

Chapter 6

Involving Children and Young People in their Own Care

The Midlands Young Advisors

Introduction

The Midlands Young Advisors were formed in 2017 as part of the Children and Young People's Improving Access to Psychological Therapies (CYP IAPT) initiative. The team consists of up to 14 children and young people aged between 16 and 25, based in the Midlands region, with experiences of mental health challenges, service access, and/or a passion for improving children and young people's mental health services. We advocate for the importance of including children and young people at the centre of their care and to ensure their voices are heard, taken into consideration, and acted upon, in a non-tokenistic way. Our work spans a variety of tasks, including, but not limited to: lived experience talks and consultancy, creating and delivering training for children and young people, parents, and mental health professionals, running engagement groups, and conducting research. This chapter has been written by a number of the team and includes a combination of our individual and group lived experiences, while also building upon existing research.

The statement, 'involving children and young people in their own care' might at first appear almost self-explanatory: how would it be possible to care for someone *without* them being part of it or affected by it? Perhaps here it is useful to refocus our definition of 'involve' away from being passively affected and instead to consider the idea of involvement as inclusion and actively taking part (Cambridge Dictionary 2022).

This approach recognises that the person accessing services holds expertise around what works for them, and how these solutions need to be approached (Health Education England [HEE] 2017; Health Innovation Network 2017). It recognises that the wants, needs, hopes, and dreams of a child and young person are paramount when deciding the best course of action for said child or young person. Ultimately, those on the receiving end of this care are the experts, and it is vital they are placed at the centre of their recovery journey. This is echoed by guidelines, such as the NHS Act (2006), which states that clinical commissioning groups have a

DOI: 10.4324/9781003288800-6

responsibility for promoting the involvement of each individual, and their carers or representatives, in decision-making relating to their care and treatment. Furthermore, more recently the NHS Long Term Plan (2019) stated the need for patients to receive more person-centred care, and for greater involvement from and choices for those accessing services. If you wish to read more about this statutory duty to involve young people in their own care, the introductory chapter covers this in greater detail.

By taking this definition, involving children and young people in their own care would not have one standardised form in which it takes place. It is instead, that during the entire process of engaging with a child or young person, focus should be placed on their needs, and keeping the service user at the core of any decision-making. Ultimately, how this looks may differ dependent on each situation or individual, and it is accepting that there is no 'one size fits all' but rather, finding what fits each person individually is the best way forward.

This chapter, written by young people themselves, adopts the view that involving an individual in their own care in a way that prioritises their wants, needs, hopes, and dreams, can be referred to as 'person-centred care'. The majority of content discussed within this chapter will relate specifically to the context of children and young people's mental health services.

We begin by outlining what person-centred care is and how it may look, followed by looking at some of the benefits and challenges when implementing person-centred care. The latter proportion of the chapter continues by considering examples and tools that may be useful for implementing person-centred care, and provides some recommendations for person-centred care. To do this, we will be drawing on a mixture of theoretical developments, best practice, and expertise by experience to form a comprehensive overview of what it means to involve children and young people in their own care, and ways which we can ensure this is being done throughout services.

What is person-centred care?

We begin this chapter by putting forward our own definition of person-centred care within children and young people's mental health services:

> Person-centred care is an approach which involves professionals and service providers working collaboratively with those accessing the service, in order to ensure the care being provided suits the needs and aspirations of a child or young person and their recovery.

This person-centred approach begins to remove rigid boundaries and ways of working with children and young people, and enables service users the voice to communicate what support it is that they need: How are we to know what would be of most benefit to an individual within their care without asking them first and involving them in this process? Therefore, the person experiencing mental distress and accessing a service must always be at the forefront of every collective decision made. In doing this, we can also proactively prompt recovery, as person-centred care enables children and young people to enhance and reclaim their 'own' sense of recovery (Hall et al. 2013). Services and service providers should empower young people to engage in conversations about their care, and particularly their preferences and needs, to encourage discussions generally about mental health whilst also enabling young people to take ownership of their journey through services.

In order for a truly person-centred approach to be adopted, a professional mindset shift may also be beneficial. Service providers should begin to see their role as being more focused on this empowerment of the young person, and striving towards jointly figuring out solutions rather than directing the child or young person what to do. It will involve a change in the typical style of interaction with a service user, from a traditionally paternalistic style, to a more collaborative approach, which involves shared decision-making (Gask and Coventry 2012).

What do young people think when they hear the words 'person-centred care'?

We asked a group of young people what came to their minds when they thought about person-centred care and what this might look like, these were their answers:

- Understanding and being open to non-traditional conversations relating to well-being, such as the link between mind, body, and soul.
- Asking for feedback about a service and actually taking this on board, and communicating with the service user in the process.
- Attempting to reduce stigma and creating a safe space for individuals to openly discuss their thoughts and feelings.
- Taking a holistic approach to involving young people in every aspect of their care.
- Not assuming one size fits all!
- Involving those aged 12 and under where appropriate, but altering the ways in which this involvement is facilitated to ensure meaningful engagement.
- Considering a variety of alternative ways to support an individual and asking them what works for their needs.
- Having a service whereby staff no longer feel solely responsible for the young person's outcome, but where the process is seen as collaborative and a shared-journey.

- Having a service where pathways are not rigid or prescribed, or whereby the focus is not on 'fixing' an individual, but working with them to reach their goal.
- Involving the young person every step of the way, including in the referral and discharge process.
- Adapting the methods of communication or service delivery to a way that fits with the service user and their needs.
- Open and honest communication with the service users about expectations and realities.
- Involving young people in the assessment and diagnosis process, and also understanding when achieving a diagnosis may or may not be helpful for a young person.
- Not assuming all young people don't know their needs, but empowering them to discover themselves further and understand how these needs can be met.
- Understanding and respecting the service user's wishes, where possible, about how and when information relating to their care is shared.

One young person in particular expressed that to them, person-centred care is 'highly specific and personalised', and involves having a care plan which is 'coproduced with them, and the care itself is about empowering a young person to set their own goals and to take steps towards their own recovery'. They further shared that a service providers role is to 'give them evidence-based support based on their own actions and achievements' and to help them 'find their sense of self and embrace their identity'. This individual highlights the importance of person-centred care in creating a safe space in which a young person feels free and able to form goals and embrace their identity.

Link to participation

When asked about person-centred care, one young person shared how they felt the core values of this approach overlap with those of participation. They shared how both participation and person-centred care are about 'letting the lived experience of the service user/prospective service user have an influence on how care is experienced'. Both aim to empower service users, and widen the conversation about service delivery, so input is more mutual and less hierarchical between the traditional 'professionals' and those with the valuable lived experience. It also isn't the case that the service user should 'solely dictate their own care' but that their perspective should be 'equally valued'.

When adopting the principles of participation and person-centred care, a service begins creating a culture which actively seeks to hear the voices of those impacted by a service, and it changes the narrative from what needs to be done to fix a situation, to what could be done to support someone to achieve their ideal scenario. This culture begins to place an emphasis on opening up the conversation about potential ways a service can be provided, or improved, and avoiding jumping to conclusions or making decisions on someone else's behalf. Particularly within mental health care, there is often an over-reliance on diagnosis, and an assumption that the end goal is symptom erasure. However, a person-centred approach looks for what the service user is seeking support for, what a meaningful quality of life is for them, and then working together to move towards that.

Furthermore, both participation and person-centred care encourage service users to identify areas of difficulty or where they feel there are struggles, and allows them to find solutions or smaller goals, which can help. For example, in the case of outcome measurement, it is important to include young people and their families in this process. This can be through collaborating on the design and development of outcome measurement tools, to ensure they are truly representative of the outcomes young people think are of most importance (Moran et al. 2012). This can also be through understanding how different young people may feel the application of these tools would be most beneficial. Using outcome measures "needs to be a more collaborative process", so service users and services are aiming towards the same goal and measuring progress in the same way (Moran et al. 2012: 65). By placing the young people's voices at the centre of services, and offering them opportunities to shape the way these services run, services are able to constantly evolve and develop in a way that benefits service users' recovery.

Benefits and challenges

Placing the service user at the centre of their treatment and allowing children and young people to make informed decisions about their care from referral to discharge carries a number of benefits for that young person. It also causes a direct, knock-on effect that subsequently benefits those close to the young person, in both a personal and professional setting. Think of a young person's care team and personal support network as a machine built up of many mechanical cogs. At the core of this mechanism lies one central cog, the young person, whose rotation triggers the rotation of every other cog. Without this cog, the mechanism does not rotate or move at all and, similarly, increasing the efficacy of this central cog, increases the efficacy of the mechanism as a whole. If a young person is able to fully reap the benefits of the care and treatment offered to them, every 'stakeholder', be it personal or professional, in the young person's recovery will also benefit. See Figure 6.1 for a visualisation of the 'cog model'.

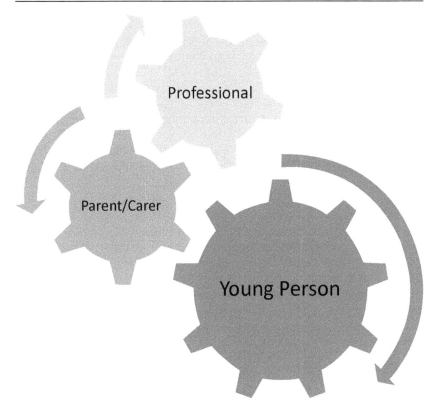

Figure 6.1 The 'cog model'

When attempting to fully involve young people within their own care, barriers and obstacles arise due to natural hierarchies, systems engrained within services, and anxieties from the service users. It is important to recognise that these systemic barriers exist and we can only find methods that address and overcome them once we have accepted both their presence and the reasoning behind their existence. Think back to our cog model, for example, and imagine that the mechanism becomes jammed. Without knowing the cause of the sudden standstill, one would have to take the entire mechanism apart, rebuilding it from scratch and hoping they eliminate the initial cause at some point within this process. However, if they are already aware of the issues that may occur in the running of the mechanism, these can be directly targeted prior to even starting the machine, reducing the likelihood of reaching that same standstill. Furthermore, if the mechanism does still jam despite preventative action, the likely causes of this malfunction are already known, so repair may be far easier as the issue can be localised to the problem areas rather than dismantling the whole system. In order to fully understand how this mechanism of care can be improved from involving young people, it is first important to understand what each stake-holder stands to gain, individually, from this involvement and the obstacles that may prevent that involvement from occurring.

Young person

Central to this mechanism of care, young people accessing mental health services for the first time can often feel overwhelmed and intimidated by what is often a new and unfamiliar environment. From the moment a child or young person receives a referral; the amount of information regarding their treatment, and the ability the young person has to be involved holistically within their own care, will shape their recovery process. Care that does not allow the receiver to have their voice heard at every stage often leaves the young person feeling out of control and like a passive actor in their recovery journey. With some studies linking feelings of lack of autonomy and agency to the development of mental health challenges (Wiersma et al. 2011), it is important that as much is done as possible to reduce this feeling. Facilitating service-user involvement within their own care, and wider service development, can help children and young people to regain an element of control over their mental health outcomes. Secondly, those individuals with multiple needs, or those with a low level of knowledge and skills around support options and managing mental health, may benefit greatly from the ability to receive information regarding their care. This allows service users to make informed decisions surrounding their care to gain a greater understanding of their difficulties and develop more self-awareness, and to reduce feelings of isolation as they have greater awareness of the support network surrounding them. They can therefore have choice in their care options and feel fully integrated in decision-making conversations, creating a higher quality of care delivered, with better outcomes for those who traditionally would have less flexible treatment plans (Forder et al. 2012). In fact, young people who have active involvement within their own care planning tend to both report greater satisfaction with the care that they received and experience less regret about the decisions they have been supported to make (Redding 2016) and treatment tends to be more informed and based on personal preference (Coulter et al. 2015; Da Silva 2012). This strongly supports person-centred, participative care.

One key obstacle that children and young people may face regarding involvement in their own care is a lack of awareness and knowledge surrounding treatment areas, and available support. As pointed out by a young person in the following publication:

> When it comes to what I'm actually supposed to do to treat whatever ailment I have, [my GP] doesn't explain it that well.
>
> (MeFirst n.d.)

In other areas of the healthcare services, such as physical health or dental health, there are often clear, established pathways that an individual can follow to access treatment or support. However, within children and young people's mental health services, these set pathways don't always exist. Often, there are multiple, different services available to young people, and a variety of different ways of referral to these services. Furthermore, symptoms are generally less salient and often require further exploration, and the experiences of one individual with a specific mental health difficulty are not always the same as another individual with the same diagnosis. A physical health issue usually has clear indicators of improvement, such as a decrease in pain or increase in usual function. Mental health issues, however, are not this cut and dry when it comes to recovery. Although progress can be measured through tools such as outcome measures, these are subjective and not always completely accurate.

Furthermore, there is often a range of support or treatment options made accessible to young people in order to lessen the impact that their symptoms have on their day-to-day life, varying from medication, to talking therapies, through to electroconvulsive therapy. Yet, if young people are not actively engaged in services, service providers may therefore not truly understand the difficulties each young person is having and may not have collaborative discussions about these available treatment options and the service user's recovery goals. This excludes young people from decisions surrounding their care, and also limits the ability for young people step up and voice their opinions, as they are not provided with the knowledge needed to enable them to do this. It is, therefore, imperative that young people are provided with the information, using language that they are familiar with and understand, as to what support pathways are available, from the moment they enter a service. This will help to ensure young people are appropriately informed to go on to make decisions regarding their own care. Informed choices are vital when considering person-centred care, and empowering young people to take ownership over their recovery.

Parents/carers

Carers and/or parents report how important it is that they feel informed around their young person's care and are also valued as an 'expert' about their child (Iachini et al. 2015). Young Minds state:

> Parents/carers have a wealth of information about their child/young person and on this basis form part of any solution. Without [services] listening to us and our young people you risk making huge assumptions about care needed.

> (Young Minds, n.d.)

Evidence also demonstrates that having involvement from parents or carers in a young person's mental health recovery can be incredibly beneficial for a young person's outcomes, as well as for the parent or carer (Oruche et al. 2014). When young people are placed at the centre of their care, these conversations around involving their carer in their recovery journey can be done in a way which meets their needs. Parents and carers can join in on this process of achieving a shared goal, but in a way that is guided by the young person's wishes. The person-centred care approach empowers young people to take ownership of their recovery, and therefore enable them to openly share this information with their carers if they wish. By creating this environment of open communication, young people may feel more likely to engage in this conversation with their parents or carers.

This positive involvement of parents and carers, in a way that is welcomed by the young person, also empowers parents and carers to support their child and provide a different perspective and insight into the young person's difficulties, which can be incredibly helpful when it comes to the shared decision-making process (Bjønness et al. 2022). Furthermore, parents, carers, and family form a crucial part of an individual's support system and have the potential to have a significant impact on an individual's recovery (Tew et al. 2012).

Therefore, when parents and carers are able to have a level of involvement in the young person's mental healthcare, and as a family can identify ways to support their loved one, this is only going to positively impact their recovery (Waller et al. 2018). Additionally, in our opinion, involving parents and carers in a meaningful and positive way means they are less likely to feel isolated or disconnected from that young person's recovery journey, and therefore will be more likely to adopt a supportive and healthy mindset towards the service and the young person's care.

The feelings on this of a young person are highlighted below:

> When they talk to my parents instead of me, I can't understand what they're saying because my parents are adults, and I can't understand the words they're saying. If they were talking to me, they would use easier words.
>
> (MeFirst n.d.)

This high level of investment from parents/carers can, however, create a barrier between a young person and the professional or clinician providing their care. At times, young people have reported how it felt as though their parent or carer was the one being prioritised when they were accessing mental healthcare (Harper et al. 2013). Professionals may also tend to view parents and carers as the more mature and knowledgeable member of the mechanism and may begin to treat the young person like a child who has no autonomy, and all communications will be aimed towards the parent or carer (Harper et al. 2013). This may be done through using language directed at the parent or carer, such as clinical terms, which can often be inaccessible to young people. Particularly in instances where a young person does not have a solid understanding of their condition or care options, this would further isolate them from engaging in their care planning. This is where the mechanism in the 'cog model' begins to fail as it no longer focuses on the young person at the centre, but instead the parent or carer. Furthermore, some young people do not wish to have their parents or carers involved in their care, and when implementing person-centred care, it is important to acknowledge this where possible, rather than ignoring the wishes of the young person (Gibson et al. 2016).

From our experience as young people who have accessed mental health services, it is quite often incredibly anxiety provoking when engaging with authority figures, such as your mental healthcare providers, which makes it hard to challenge instances when your needs are not being met or considered. Furthermore, some young people report that having a parent or carer in their sessions with them leads to self-censorship, where they feel unable to speak openly (Coyne et al. 2006). This means that the cycle of dampening the young person's voice, and instead listening to the parent/carer's voice, may continue. The relationship therefore builds between the professional and parent/carer, and not between the professional and young person, isolating the young person further. The parent or carer, however, is not always the expert relating to how the young person is coping, or the treatment that would be most beneficial to that young person. So, focusing on the parent's or carer's voice rather than the young person can lead to the young person feeling isolated and disengaged from their care, but also the development of a care plan that is likely to not be truly addressing their needs and therefore not effectively aiding that young person's recovery.

Professionals

Professionals are key in delivering a person-centred approach that will provide a greater standard of care that is more likely to target the needs of the service user. This will in-turn benefit them, as professionals, as they experience the accompanying benefits of this more effective service. In using a person-centre approach, members of a service user's care team are able to gain an in-depth understanding of the service user's struggles, and therefore the areas they may benefit from having support, whilst also achieving a greater sense of job satisfaction. Clinicians are also able to build a higher level of trust and rapport with clients when involving young people in care through processes such as shared decision-making (Abrines-Jaume et al.

2014). This increased trust and strength of relationship between service user and provider has a direct impact on both parties' approach to the service. Service providers and professionals working within Children and Young People's (CYPs) mental health services, are more likely to be able to see a direct positive impact of their work with a young person, increasing their ability to remain understanding, as well as increasing real and meaningful communication between service user and provider. This communication is cited by staff within healthcare roles as being crucial to the success of their role (Institute for Healthcare Communication 2011) and so are essential qualities to be able to optimise when working with a young person and their support network. Leading to the argument that services as a whole could be able to cut costs and wait times when centering a service user within their own treatment plan.

Processes and features of a service that allow a service user to access support in the way that is most comfortable for them, increases the likelihood that the user will attend appointments and engage with care (Ansell et al. 2017). This decrease in costs and wait times is also the case because young people are able to verbalise their exact needs and expectations from their care and as such, assumptions being made on their behalf are minimised, reducing wasted time and resources. If communication is direct and clear between user and provider, treatment can be planned in accordance with the needs of the service user, and their recovery can be monitored with increased accuracy, so alterations to their care plan can be made promptly where necessary.

One obstacle that professionals may face when trying to implement person-centred care is that external factors could impact their ability to provide said care in the first place. For example, at the time of writing this text, services were still dealing with the backlog and increase of cases of those children and young people requiring access to mental health services due to the COVID-19 pandemic. When events like this occur, not only does this impact the capacity of service providers and their ability to give each caseload their full attention, but it can also lead to burnout. This professional burnout is likely to detract from a practitioner's passion and the likelihood of person-centred care being a top priority decreases rapidly (Morse et al. 2011; Salyers et al. 2016). This is where this culture shift, from person-centred care being an additional element to a service, to fully integrating person-centred care approaches and participation within every aspect of a service is crucial. If something becomes so engrained in the everyday, it will maintain a priority when these constraints begin to tighten. In order to achieve this culture shift though, it is also important to have the whole of the workforce on board with these initiatives, including commissioners and other staff members who may not necessarily work directly with service users. It is this holistic shift to placing young people at the heart of services that will make a difference.

Additionally, there is also often a power imbalance between the service users and practitioners or professionals (Bee et al. 2015). This imbalance may be created due to the presence of one individual who is considered an expert in the field of mental health, the professional, and an individual who may know little to nothing on the subject (the young person) and may be heightened due to the obvious age difference. This assumed power imbalance can lead to a young person feeling very ostracised from their practitioner, and the service as a whole (Gharabaghi 2013; Harper et al. 2013). It is important to note that this imbalance is very often not the fault of the practitioner, but it is essential to recognise that it exists in order to minimise its effects. In recognising its existence, professionals can work to counteract it, building a firmer working relationship with the young person, and allowing the necessary open two-way dialogue to remain uninhibited. A young person must not only feel understood, but respected and comfortable in order for them to involve themselves within their care. Establishing this mutual, non-judgemental working relationship, in which communication, trust, and respect goes both ways, can result in greater engagement from the young person.

This section has demonstrated some of the various benefits and challenges of person-centred care, and how this impacts not only the young person accessing the service, but also the service providers and parents or carers. We acknowledge that whilst person-centred care has many benefits, there are challenges and barriers that often prevent it from taking place. However, by addressing these barriers, and discussing why they take place and the impact they have on those within the mechanism of care, we can begin to think of ways around them. We now want to take a look at some practical ways of implementing a person-centred care approach, and where we can begin to look at how we can practically overcome these hurdles.

Tools for person-centred care

With such diverse and divergent approaches to supporting individuals with mental health difficulties, the journey to find support that 'works' can be frustrating and bewildering. However, as we have discussed, person-centred care can not only facilitate an easier discovery of what support works best (as it takes guidance from the immediate wants and needs of the young person) but also offers a methodology that can be drawn upon across mental health disciplines. One way to embed this child- and young-person focused ideology is through the creation of person-centred tools in mental health care. In accordance with our earlier definition, to be person-centred is to recognise:

- Children and young people should be active participants within their own care and support.

- Each child and young person holds the unique expertise of what works for them, rooted within their wants, needs, hopes, and personal background.
- Person-centred approaches are not focused around the standardising of outcomes (e.g., the same support for everyone) but on processes (e.g., all children and young people are given the same opportunities and empowerment to draw upon their unique expertise to create a pathway of support that works best for them).

As such, any tools for person-centred care would be a standard template, process, or practice that meaningfully draws upon the expertise of the supported person (the child or young person) in an act of collaborative support. Given the fluctuating and ever-developing nature of what tools are considered 'best practice', and in order to delve more deeply into what constitutes as a beneficial person-centred tool, this section will not aim to complete an exhaustive exploration of all available tools. Instead, it will critically analyse the Wellness Recovery Action Plan as an example tool in order to unearth the possible strengths, implementation difficulties, and areas of consideration needed when creating a person-centred tool.

The Wellness Recovery Action Plan (WRAP) is a person-centred tool that offers individuals the opportunity to document what works for looking after their mental health, both for their personal use and for the reference of mental health practitioners. It was designed by Mary Ellen Copeland and Jane Winterling in response to the demand for a way to organise well-being tools and strategies used by those living with mental health challenges (Copeland, 2002; The Copeland Center for Wellness and Recovery, 2020). The WRAP considers personal values and approaches to good well-being, what a difficult day can look like and what can support the management of this, as well as how the individual can be empowered and supported through the process of crisis, from beginning to end. It can be broken down into three key sections, each exploring a different moment in one's recovery and what is felt is most needed, in regards to support, by that individual (Figure 6.1). Benefits may vary, but Mak et al.'s (2022) study showed the potential for the use of WRAPs to lead to improvements in participants' rates of depressive symptoms, anxiety symptoms, feelings of hope and empowerment, and personal recovery. Here we can see how providing support that is person-centred does not just lead to benefits in well-being, but it assists with the motivation and belief in their recovery, which in turn will enhance the benefits seen.

Wellness Recovery Action Plan example content:

1 Daily maintenance

Example prompts
- What do I need to do/avoid to stay well?
- What does a good/bad day look like for me?
- What are my triggers and how can I manage these?

2 Crisis plan

Example prompts
- How can I tell I am in crisis?
- Who do I want contacting and what support do I want from them?
- Who (individuals, e.g., relatives or professionals, or organisations, e.g., hospitals) do I not want involved in my support?
- Who is currently involved in my care and how to contact?
- What medication do I take and what alternatives would I prefer if unavailable?

3 Post-crisis plan

Example prompts
- How can I tell I am no longer in crisis?
- What support will I need while coming out of crisis?
- How can I tell that I am ready to return to my daily maintenance plan?
- What have I learnt through my crisis that I will use to change/ redevelop my WRAP?

Critical analysis of WRAP: Strengths

- Concerns what works for the CYP.
- CYP-centred language e.g., 'What do I need?', 'for me' etc.
- Does not prescribe a one-size-fits-all approach and instead empowers each child and young person to find their own solution.
- Places CYP at the centre, e.g., the child or young person is asked what support would help.
- It draws on strengths and skills, rather than assuming ineptitude or that the child or young person needs saving.
- Answers are not required for all sections.

Critical analysis of WRAP: Weaknesses

- It relies on CYP having motivation and self-belief, which can be hard to find in moments of hopelessness.

- Crisis considerations can be overwhelming.
- It assumes a pre-existing knowledge of services and support available.
- Despite being flexible and adaptable, it assumes written documents are helpful tools for everyone.
- It depends upon a Western cultural understanding/viewpoint.

Drawn upon from Crimmings (2013), Deci (2012), and GetSelfHelp (n.d.)

From our brief look at WRAPs, we are able to acknowledge how we might begin to meaningfully implement person-centred values into our working, while holding an awareness for possible traps/obstacles. Although not specifically designed as a tool for children and young people, the WRAP places the person supported as the focal point. First and foremost, it considers each person as a unique individual and recognises there is not a 'one size fits all' solution that should be imposed. The WRAP is adaptable to the needs of the user and does not necessarily require someone to be of a certain age (dependant on how the questions are adapted and which are included). To facilitate use of the tool with children and young people however, it is key to collaborate with professionals who can explain what options are available and what this looks like for the person supported. This offers a way to overcome the obstacle of lack of understanding, and studies have shown that being taught how to prepare a WRAP can feel like 'a life changing experience' (Higgins et al. 2011: 2427). As such, we can note that person-centred tools require person-centred approaches: the tool and support given must be responsive to the needs and perspective of the child or young person. If not, we risk a misunderstanding that can be read as a lack of care by children and young people, which can result in disengagement, resistance, and even defiance.

Going forward, there are many key points to take away from this chapter. The question is: how do we include young people in their care? Professionals, involved directly or indirectly with delivering services to young people, have a shared responsibility to ensure that each and every young person's voice is heard and taken on board. The outcomes for service users, and the overall experience of a service, can be improved by adopting a holistic approach to their care which places the service user right at the centre. This person-centred care approach, according to the Midlands Young Advisors, involves 'professionals and service providers working collaboratively with those accessing a service, in order to ensure the care being provided suits the needs, and aspirations of a child or young person and their recovery'. Furthermore, actively promoting participation and the wider involvement of young people within service development or decisions is just as crucial when making sure services designed for young people, and are actually representative of how young people want their care to look. Finding out what works best for young people, and what doesn't, can improve outcomes on an individual basis, as well as improving experiences for those young people yet to access services. By looking at what young people want in their care and from services on the whole, and by talking to and actively including young people in their decision making, a service becomes more well-informed and better equipped to guide young people through their recovery journeys. This recovery journey can be based off what young people want, rather than rigid, 'one size fits all' service provisions, ultimately achieving better outcomes.

Conclusion

This chapter has outlined that there are not only benefits for the service user when person-centred care is adopted, but also benefits for professionals and parents/carers of the young person accessing services. By placing young people as the centre-cog in their care, and ensuring the system is running in a way that meets their needs, the professionals and parents/carers also included in this system begin to thrive and work around the young person effectively. It is important to recognise the journey to recovery is about collaboration between all parties, but that the service user is ultimately the expert when it comes to understanding their wants, desires, and needs. This isn't to say the young person should completely dictate their own care or service provisions, but that they should hold an equally valued perspective. This shared decision-making can also reduce power imbalances which can at times leave young people feeling disempowered within their own care, ultimately leading to disengagement. It is for the professional to counteract this feeling, by ensuring the young person has some element of control over their care, and by helping them to understand the options about the direction in which their care can go. Making decisions for a young person only creates further power imbalance, and clinicians should work *with* the young person not *on* them.

Challenges such as neutralising this power imbalance, and ensuring parents/carers aren't taking over a young person's care, are inevitable when providing mental health support to children and young people. However, it is the ways in which services respond to these challenges that are vital. Through implementing person-centred care and elements of participation across a service, in all areas that impact a young person's care, a culture can be created which emphasises the service user as an equally valid member in decision-making. But also creating a safe space whereby open communication is encouraged, and inclusivity is a high priority, creates an environment in which young people thrive and feel empowered to become more invested in, and take greater responsibility for, their own care. This inclusivity within mental health support for young people can look like: offering choices of care pathways and providing information which allows for informed decision making, asking what goals a young person has and is collaboratively working towards these, or just getting to know a young person outside of their mental health difficulties.

Ultimately, person-centred care should be a fundamental element of young people's mental health services, as the wants, needs, hopes, and dreams of a child or young person are paramount when considering their pathway to recovery, and living a happy, fulfilled life.

With thanks to Abi Banham, Melek Andrews, Harry Dixon, Lewis Lockwood, Amber Jackson, Oli Hawley, and Bry Hodgetts for their work on this chapter.

If you wish to read more about the Midlands Young Advisor team, please go to https://associatedevelopmentsolutions.com/the-midlands-young-advisors/ to get an overview of the work we do, as well as having a look at some graphics designed by the team to summarise the key recommendations from this chapter and some quotes gathered directly from children and young people.

References

Abrines-Jaume, N., Midgley, N., Hopkins, K., Hoffman, J., Martin, K., Law, D. and Wolpert, M. (2014). A qualitative analysis of implementing shared decision making in Child and Adolescent Mental Health Services in the United Kingdom: Stages and facilitators. *Clinical Child Psychology and Psychiatry*, 21(1), 19–31, doi:10.1177/1359104514547596.

Ansell, D., Crispo, J. A. G., Simard, B. and Bjerre, L. M. (2017). Interventions to reduce wait times for primary care appointments: A systematic review. *BMC Health Services Research*, 17(1), doi:10.1186/s12913-017-2219-y.

Bee, P., Price, O., Baker, J. and Lovell, K. (2015). Systematic synthesis of barriers and facilitators to service user-led care planning. *British Journal of Psychiatry*, 207(2), 104–114, doi:10.1192/bjp.bp.114.152447.

Bjønness, S., Grønnestad, T., Johannessen, J. O. and Storm, M. (2022). Parents' perspectives on user participation and shared decision-making in adolescents' inpatient mental healthcare. *Health Expectations*. doi:10.1111/hex.13443.

Cambridge Dictionary (2022). Involve. [Online] Available at: https://dictionary.cambridge.org/dictionary/english/involve [Accessed 20 July 2022].

The Copeland Center for Wellness and Recovery (2020). History of WRAP. https://copelandcenter.com/what-wrap/history-wrap [Accessed 2 July 2022].

Copeland, M. E. (2002). Wellness recovery action plan: A system for monitoring, reducing and eliminating uncomfortable or dangerous physical symptoms and emotional feelings. *Occupational Therapy in Mental Health*, 17(3–4), 127–150, doi:10.1300/J004v17n03_09.

Coulter, A., Entwistle, V. A., Eccles, A., Ryan, S., Shepperd, S. and Perera, R. (2015). Personalised care planning for adults with chronic or long-term health conditions. *Cochrane Database of Systematic Reviews*. [Online] 3(3). doi:10.1002/14651858.cd010523.pub2.

Coyne, I. T., Hayes, E., Gallagher, P. and Regan, G. (2006). *Giving Children a Voice: Investigation of Children's Experiences of Participation in Consultation and Decision-making in Irish Hospitals*. Dublin: Office of the Minister for Children.

Crimmings, C. (2013). A guide to completing your Wellness Recovery Action Plan (WRAP). St Vincent's Mental Health Service, Acute Inpatient Service. https://healthsciences.unimelb.edu.au/__data/assets/pdf_file/0006/3391719/Guide-to-developing-a-WRAP-for-acute-inpatient-service-and-for-community-settings.pdf [Accessed 2 July 2022].

Da Silva, D. (2012). Helping people share decision making. [Online] Available at: https://www.health.org.uk/publications/helping-people-share-decision-making.

Deci, E. (2012). Promoting motivation, health, and excellence. Available at: https://tedxflourcity.com/?q=speaker/2012/ed-deci [Accessed 7 July 2022].

Forder, J., Jones, K., Glendinning, C., Caiels, J., Welch, E., Baxter, K., Davidson, J. and Windle, K. (2012). Evaluation of the personal health budget pilot programme. [Online] Available at: https://www.york.ac.uk/inst/spru/research/pdf/phbe.pdf.

Gask, L. and Coventry, P. (2012). Person-centred mental health care: The challenge of implementation. *Epidemiology and Psychiatric Sciences*. [Online] 21(2), 139–144. doi:10.1017/s2045796012000078.

GetSelfHelp. (n.d.). The Wellness Recovery Action Plan, 'WRAP'. https://www.getselfhelp.co.uk/docs/WRAP.pdf [Accessed 2 July 2022].

Gharabaghi, K. (2013). *Professional Issues in Child and Youth Care Practice*. 1st ed. Hoboken: Taylor and Francis, 75–76.

Gibson, K., Cartwright, C., Kerrisk, K., Campbell, J. and Seymour, F. (2016). What young people want: A qualitative study of adolescents' priorities for engagement across psychological services. *Journal of Child and Family Studies*, 25(4), 1057–1065. doi:10.1007/s10826-015-0292-6.

Hall, A., Wren, M. and Kirby, S. D. (2013). Care planning in mental health: Promoting recovery. 2nd edition. ed. *The Open Library*. Chichester, West Sussex, UK: John Wiley & Sons Inc. Available at: https://openlibrary.org/books/OL31143576M/Care_planning_in_mental_health [Accessed 10 June 2022].

Harper, B., Dickson, J. M. and Bramwell, R. (2013). Experiences of young people in a 16–18 Mental Health Service. *Child and Adolescent Mental Health*, 19(2), 90–96. doi:10.1111/camh.12024.

Health Education England (HEE) (2017). Person-centred Care. [Online] Health Education England. Available at: https://www.hee.nhs.uk/our-work/person-centred-care.

Health Innovation Network. (2017). What is Person-Centred Care and Why is it Important? [online] Available at: https://healthinnovationnetwork.com/system/ckeditor_assets/attachments/41/what_is_person-centred_care_and_why_is_it_important.pdf.

Higgins, A. *et al.* (2011) Evaluation of mental health recovery and wellness recovery action planning in Ireland: A mixed methods pre-post evaluation. *Journal of Advanced Nursing*, 68(11), 2418–2428.

Iachini, A. L., Hock, R. M., Thomas, M. and Clone, S. (2015). Exploring the youth and parent perspective on practitioner behaviors that promote treatment engagement. *Journal of Family Social Work*, 18 (1), 57–73. doi:10.1080/ 10522158.2014.974293.

Institute for Healthcare Communication (2011). Impact of communication in healthcare. [Online] Healthcarecomm.org. Available at: https://healthcarecomm. org/about-us/impact-of-communication-in-healthcare/.

Mak, W. W. S., Tsoi, E. W. S. and Wong, H. C. Y. (2022). Brief Wellness Recovery Action Planning (WRAP®) as a mental health self-management tool for community adults in Hong Kong: A randomized controlled trial. *Journal of Mental Health*, 1–8. https://doi.org/10.1080/09638237.2022.2069723.

MeFirst (n.d.). What are the barriers and challenges? [Online] Available at: http s://www.mefirst.org.uk/why/what-are-the-barriers-challenges/.

Moran, P., Kelesidi, K., Guglani, S., Davidson, S. and Ford, T. (2012). What do parents and carers think about routine outcome measures and their use? A focus group study of CAMHS attenders. *Clinical Child Psychology and Psychiatry*. [Online] 17(1), 65–79. doi:10.1177/1359104510391859.

Morse, G., Salyers, M. P., Rollins, A. L., Monroe-DeVita, M. and Pfahler, C. (2011). Burnout in mental health services: A review of the problem and its remediation. *Administration and Policy in Mental Health and Mental Health Services Research*, 39(5), 341–352. https://doi.org/10.1007/s10488-011-0352-1.

NHS Act 2006 (2006). c41, https://www.legislation.gov.uk/ukpga/2006/41/contents.

NHS Long Term Plan (2019). The NHS long term plan. Available at: https:// www.longtermplan.nhs.uk/.

Oruche, U. M., Downs, S., Holloway, E., Draucker, C., and Aalsma, M. (2013). Barriers and facilitators to treatment participation by adolescents in a community mental health clinic. *Journal of Psychiatric and Mental Health Nursing*, 21(3), 241–248. https://doi.org/10.1111/jpm.12076.

Redding, D. (2016). New approaches to value in health and care. [Online] Available at: http://www.health.org.uk/publications/new-approaches-to-value-in-hea lth-and-care.

Salyers, M. P., Bonfils, K. A., Luther, L., Firmin, R. L., White, D. A., Adams, E. L. and Rollins, A. L. (2016). The relationship between professional burnout and quality and safety in healthcare: A meta-analysis. *Journal of General Internal Medicine*, 32(4), 475–482. doi:10.1007/s11606-016-3886-9.

Tew, J., Ramon, S., Slade, M., Bird, V., Melton, J. and Le Boutillier, C. (2012). Social factors and recovery frommental health difficulties: A review of the evidence. *British Journal of Social Work*, 42, 443–460.

Waller, S., Reupert, A., Ward, B., McCormick, F. and Kidd, S. (2018). Family-focused recovery: Perspectives from individuals with a mental illness. *International Journal of Mental Health Nursing*, 28(1), 247–255. doi:10.1111/inm.12528.

Wiersma, J. E., van Oppen, P., van Schaik, D. J. F., van der Does, A. J. W., Beekman, A.T.F. and Penninx, B.W.J.H. (2011). Psychological characteristics of chronic depression: A longitudinal cohort study. *The Journal of Clinical Psychiatry*, 72(3) 288–294. https://doi.org/10.4088/ JCP.09m05735blu.

Young Minds (n.d.) Evolving by involving. [Online] Available at: https://www.youngm inds.org.uk/media/0lcbhmqd/evolving-by-involving.pdf [Accessed 9 June 2022].

Chapter 7

A Guide to Parent and Carer Participation

Wendy Minhinnett (She/Her) and
Nikki Chapman (She/Her)

Our Stories

My first encounter with services went something like this:

> What support can you offer me?
> > Parent of a young person experiencing mental
> > health difficulties

> None, we support the child, you need to go to the GP for
> Counselling.
> > Children and Young People's Mental Health
> > (CYPMH) Professional

Counselling was not what I needed, not at that point anyway. However, I followed the professional's advice, got an appointment with a counsellor at my GP surgery and after pouring my heart and soul out they couldn't provide what I needed either. What I did need at that time was practical advice, information, and involvement in my daughter's care so I could better understand and know how to help. I was desperate; my daughter was unwell, and I didn't know what to do. I've since been told by CYPMH professionals with whom I have a good relationship that I was viewed as a 'problem parent' who pushed for information and asked questions. Eventually, to meet my needs I was given some independent support from a CYPMH psychologist who helped me with ideas for how I could help my daughter. It's quite sad to look back and think that support for families was not really considered as part of the child's care at the time. Things have come a long way since then, but there is still much to do.

I now know some of the things I was doing were making things worse, but I was doing the best I could with the information and knowledge I had at the time. Thankfully our family came out the other side of these very dark times, my daughter is 24 now and living an amazing life. I set up a parent/carer support group and began working both locally and

DOI: 10.4324/9781003288800-7

nationally to help parent and carer voices be included in CYPMH services. I know we are one of the lucky families; we survived the fight, not everyone does.

Wendy Minhinnett

As adoptive parents, our child had been accessing Child and Adolescent Mental Health Services (CAMHS) off and on from a very young age. On each occasion we received great support from knowledgeable and compassionate clinicians who listened to us and included us in our child's care. We were lucky. When we read newspaper articles about how things were in other parts of the country, we came to feel even more fortunate. When those articles highlighted ever-increasing waiting times, parents desperate for support and a system 'at breaking point' we felt more than lucky – we felt like we had won the CAMHS lottery.

So, when one day we were waiting for our child's appointment and on the coffee table in front of us was a leaflet asking for parents to express their interest in a new parent participation group, I immediately felt compelled to sign up. I felt strongly that it shouldn't be about 'being lucky' and if we could have the 'CAMHS golden ticket' then other parents should have that too. I wanted to be part of making that a reality. The parent participation group was formed, and we later developed a parent support group too. We are still accessing support for our child and some days are easier than others. We will get there though; each day we get a little stronger. Knowing that I can use our experiences to help create positive change for families both locally and nationally gives me a purpose and the strength to get up again each time we get knocked down.

Nikki Chapman

©WendyMinhinnett

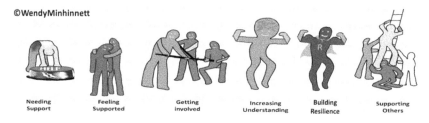

| Needing Support | Feeling Supported | Getting involved | Increasing Understanding | Building Resilience | Supporting Others |

Figure 7.1 Parent journey model – from needing support to supporting others
Source: Author.

The model is not linear, parents enter, exit and travel in both directions depending on their needs at the time.

I Needing Support

> One of the hardest things to experience is the sense of helplessness. I would happily have walked over burning coals or climbed Everest if there was even the slightest chance it would have helped my child's mental health. I desperately wanted to help my child and when nothing seemed to be working, it was like, please, just give me something, anything I can do to help.
>
> Parent

When a parent or carer first becomes concerned about their child's mental health, they often reach out to family and friends for reassurance and support. Some are lucky and find the support they were looking for, others find a lack of understanding, judgement, and even blame from those closest to them.

As parents become increasingly concerned about their child's health and have exhausted all the personal/family options available to them, they usually try to access advice that will help them help their child. There are many different places that parents reach out to e.g. online (support group, website, Facebook), face to face support group, telephone helpline, text crisis service, CYPMH service, GP, school, Mental Health Support Teams, Voluntary and Community Services, religion or faith groups, or another kind of community provision. What is available to them very much depends on where they live and what their child needs. Parents often describe the experience of seeking support as like trying to find their way through a maze: very difficult to navigate, not knowing which is the right path to take, frequently running into dead ends, such as being told:

"This isn't the right service for you."
"Your child doesn't meet the criteria."
"They're fine in school."

There are also lots of instances where parents describe being provided with pages and pages of options and resources. So many that they can't process all the information they have been given and are left not knowing where to start. This can lead to feelings of being over-whelmed. As one parent said, "So I didn't do any". It is well recognised that when a person is under stress, they are more likely to experience difficulties processing information; providing parents with a short list of support options/resources targeted to the needs of their family is far more likely to lead to better outcomes for the child/young person and the family a whole.

As a parent you have two main jobs: love your child unconditionally and keep them safe. When my child was self-harming, risk taking and attempted suicide, I felt like such a failure as a parent because I hadn't kept them safe.

Parent

It is very important to be aware that even at this early stage, parents often share how they feel guilt and blame that they are "failing" as a parent. This can be exacerbated by the parent being offered, or instructed to attend, an inappropriate parenting course (we will explore the role of parenting courses later in this chapter). In our experiences, some professionals use this stigma/parent blame as a justification for excluding parents from participating in their child's care, where others ensure that parent's voices are actively listened to. Those professionals who promote parent participation in their child's care are aware that parents may have experienced many different forms of judgement and blame before they reach their door and may be fearful of how they will treat them. These professionals will take the time to explain abbreviations and things parents don't understand (e.g. the care plan). They remember that they may see the child/young person for 1 hour a week, but the other 167 hours are down to the parent. So, if they have given the child/young person any strategies they tell the parent to enable them to support their child (and help the parent avoid inadvertently working against the strategy). Parents are not asking for the confidential information their child/young person shared, they just want practical advice and information.

I still remember being so scared to go to sleep at night in case my child harmed themselves while I slept.

Parent

I was terrified that if I went to sleep before they did, they might not be alive when I woke up.

Parent

I can remember the feeling of dread as I watched the hands on the clock going round every Friday afternoon knowing that when they reached 5 o'clock we were on our own until 9 o'clock Monday morning.

Parent

Caring for a child with mental health difficulties can be extremely distressing and, in addition to the guilt and shame, many parents describe symptoms of mental and physical exhaustion. It isn't possible to live on constant high alert, living in fear each day that your child might die, without it eventually taking a direct toll on parents' mental health. While we want to be completely clear that we never condone any clinicians/staff being treated badly, there needs to be a recognition that what is sometimes seen as parents being defiant, angry, or difficult is actually terrified parents crying out for help for their child in the only way they know how, or the only way they have left, having exhausted all other avenues of accessing support.

When taking all this into account, it's clear how it is vital that any support offered to parents is flexible and accessible. For example, running groups (online or face to face) as drop-ins rather than pre-booked sessions removes an unnecessary barrier to attendance. Most parents arrange their life around their child's mental health; they may not know until just before the group whether they are able to attend. Offering a range of support is important too, for example, some days a parent being 15 minutes from home just feels too far away to be safe. When considering barriers to attendance, focus on the local community: different groups within the community have wide-ranging views around mental health, stigma and shame – how can this awareness be utilised to ensure support is available to meet the needs of all parents and carers? For example:

- Is the face-to-face group held somewhere that wouldn't highlight why someone had been there?
- Is an interpreter available?
- If the majority of people accessing social media support groups are female, how do men prefer to access support?

There are usually two outcomes from needing support: those parents who get the support they need and may move on to the next stage of the model presented in Figure 7.1 (2: Feeling Supported) or parents who can't find the support they need. A number of parents in this position who set about developing the support themselves, e.g. developing a parent support group.

2 Feeling Supported

It was the first support group of the year and the busiest group we'd ever had. This was before the days of CAMHS operating outside office hours and for these parents it had been a season of fear, rather than joy. The clinician and I were running around trying to find more chairs for all the parents and carers that had arrived, but that isn't why I'll never forget that support group. As a mother, and then a grandmother (unrelated), shared their experiences of caring for a child who self-harmed, a woman who had joined us for the first time began to cry. When we checked in with her, she said, "They're telling my story. It's so good to know I'm not the only parent going through this."

Parent

This is why parent support is so important. This is often the first time the parent experiences a safe space to talk about their feelings. Parents may have spent hours and hours thinking about and talking about their child's feelings, emotions and wellbeing, often believing that if they can "give enough of themselves" they can somehow make everything okay. When a parent feels supported and listened to, things start to feel better.

> When you are lying awake at 3am in the morning, waiting for the sun to come up, filled with doubts. Not knowing if you have the strength to get up and do it all again. It's having hope that you can get through this and having somewhere to turn to for support when I wobble that helps me get up and face the day.

Parent

The parent might have received strategies to put in place, accessed a particular support service, received reassurance they are actually doing the right things or just simply know they are not alone. Whatever it is, it gives parents a better headspace to deal with whatever life is throwing at them. It also provides hope to keep going.

It is important to recognise that what feels supportive, and what 'the right support' looks like will be different for different people, and that's okay. For some, the idea of a support group is a wonderful opportunity for connection but for others it would be their worst nightmare. Some parents really appreciate the validation from another parent who is further down the road they are travelling on, while others need the reassurance of a professional or the knowledge the support is evidence based.

> I often see the role of our support group as being to lend parents our hope until they can be supported to find their own again.

Parent Support Group Lead

Anecdotal evidence from parents facilitating support groups across the PLACE Network (The Charlie Waller Trust, 2022) (*see Section 6: supporting others below) confirms that supporting the family to maintain hope that they will get through this time is vital.

We are still building the case and evidence as to the value of parent involvement in all aspects of CYPMH. There is one formal evaluation of a parent support group that we are aware of, Rollercoaster Family Support in County Durham (Rollercoaster family support: Mental health support: County Durham, 2022). More research is needed in this area.

3 Getting Involved

> Attending the event has made me feel valued and listened to as a parent. While going through a rough journey it has gave me strength and hope that a difference could be made to children and their families in the future.
>
> Parent

Once parents feel supported they are much more likely to get involved in participation. In fact, in our experiences, for many a natural desire for involvement arises. Emotional and mental health problems have an impact on the whole family and getting involved in work around this area makes a huge difference to parental mental health and skills. It can provide something positive at a really difficult family time and also help people heal. For many it can be life changing.

Some parents enter at this point; they may not have felt a need to seek support or were not able to access additional support and involvement opportunities can provide a door into the system. Many parents who could not access the support they needed see getting involved as an opportunity to try to make things better and protect parents coming after them from the same experiences they had.

While we recognise that some parents enter at this point, many services make the mistake of not considering the first two points on this model. One parent experienced a professional who said, "We have heard all this before, we just want ideas." These services offer involvement and then wonder why they experience parents as negative/demanding. People need to have their voice heard, to be validated, before they can move forward.

Once people have been heard, and their experiences have been validated, we have found that parents are usually keen to adopt a solution-focused approach. It's about moving away from a focus on 'what we need' to make it happen to identifying 'what we have' and how we can make things better with what you've got. There is a desire to explore what we can do about it together.

Work with people, human to human, and make time and space for parents to share their experiences and insights. Enabling parents to bring the issue to life for decision makers who listen to how it feels, and see how small adjustments make huge differences to families.

Remember: parents live in the same world as professionals! They have lived through austerity too and have a clear awareness of the lack of funding and the pressures systems are under. Just like clinicians, parents do not want to waste money on grand schemes, they want the money to be stretched as far as possible so as many children/young people can be helped as possible. We all want the same thing: for our children/young people's mental health to improve, we're just coming at things from a different perspective. In fact, parents' out-of-the-box thinking can lead to exciting innovations.

When parents are giving their time to get involved, little things like cuppas, chocolate, or fruit help people to feel valued. For parents to be truly valued though, it's vital that 'non-negotiables' are set out from the outset. An open and honest discussion about this being a two way-relationship, that requires give and take on both sides and a willingness to consider service needs and to compromise when necessary, is often a good place to start. Ensuring everyone understands the parameters/limitations they are working within and have been fully informed and prepared is important. For example, if a parent is invited to join an interview panel or focus group, has the service taken the time to ensure they know what is expected of them? Are they going to be 100% part of the process in a meaningful way, i.e. will their voice be heard and their scores be counted?

To foster meaningful participation, it is often helpful to create opportunities for people to have their voice heard in creative ways, for example using art to encourage people to share experiences.

It is also vital to recognise that getting involved will almost always lead to parents reliving and sharing many of their deeply personal, often still raw, experiences. Thought must be given as to how to respectfully involve people and how they will be supported throughout; including aftercare. Disrespecting somebody is not just about not valuing their story, but what you do with it afterwards, e.g. did the parent agree to it being shared and, if so, under what conditions? This is not like 'work' for parents even when they are being paid: they are sharing themselves, their heart, it is so personal and any disrespect/devaluing of this risks a parent feeling like their heart has been stamped on. Leaving the parent feeling crushed could cause major emotional impact to them and their family.

A parent who is involved in delivering participation training for IAPT trainees in the North West of England always ends her presentation with the following two quotes, saying, "If you remember nothing else that I've said today, if you follow these quotes when working with families you won't go too far wrong!"

Be kind whenever possible. It is always possible.

Dalai Lama

I've learned that people will forget what you said, people will forget what you did, but people will never forget how you made them feel.

Maya Angelou

4 Increasing Understanding

> Thank you this has been a fantastic help. Sessions like this are an invisible cloak of armour that will really help.
>
> Parent

When parents and carers are given information tailored to their child's and family's needs, it does help and increase understanding of their child's mental health. This increased understanding, brings a sense of calm and builds confidence because it feels like at least you have some ideas of what you can do. There is no one way to do this, whether it be through a one-to-one session with a clinician or parent peer supporter, attending training, taking part in an involvement event, attending a parent support group, reading an information leaflet or a combination, it's important that these things are offered to parents. They can increase parent's knowledge and understanding of their child's mental health, their own role in supporting their child, and the systems around them that can help.

Choice is important. If you listen to parents' voices and provide choices it gives them control over what they can access in a way and time that is right for them. Sadly, for many services, the go-to answer when parents ask for support is to ask them to attend a parenting course. While there is a place for evidence-based parenting courses in this space, this approach often feeds into the parent-blame culture. Many parents receive the message that 'they are part of the problem' rather than an integral part of the solution. This perpetuates the stigma that is often associated with parents who are supporting a child with mental health challenges, causing parents to 'shut down' and being fearful to be honest because of the shame attached.

> I thought I must be responsible; I have done something wrong. I have gone over and over life events and experiences. I felt guilty for being a single parent and not being able to afford things that might help.
>
> Parent

When skills-based training and information is offered to parents and carers; it can be life changing. It takes the focus away from your parenting in general and places it around the mental health issues. Parent 'ah ha' moments can happen when you start to understand more about your child's mental health. Taking part in courses such as understanding self-harm, coping in a crisis, understanding anxiety etc. gives the practical, hands-on information parents are looking for. Courses are even more effective when they combine lived and expert experience. Parent-to-parent peer support enables supportive conversations and connections from a lived experience perspective and helps people feel less alone. Sometimes during those 'ah ha' moments, you recognise where you are going wrong but in a supportive, non-judgemental way and that matters.

> I feel more confident and reassured about dealing with everyday support to dealing with a crisis situation.
>
> Parent

It really is a two-way process, when professionals work alongside and with families to build positive and trusting relationships it can make a huge difference. Taking the time to understand what matters to families, what they are scared of, and what their interests are allows professionals to understand more about the family as people. Professionals bringing a little of themselves to the table in this process can help also. Talking about pets, interests, and where they might have gone wrong with things in their lives helps to break down barriers and enables a connection at a human level. When this happens, difficult conversations feel less judgemental.

Many parents will openly admit they have got things wrong, but in our experiences 99% of the time parents are doing the best they can with the knowledge and information they have at the time.

> Looking back, I know at times I wasn't helping but I did what I thought was the right thing.
>
> Parent

Doing the wrong thing, for the right reason is a phrase many parents are able to see when they look back. Sometimes professionals communicate the things parents may be getting 'wrong' in a blaming, judgemental way. This is a lot less likely to happen when positive relationships are in place.

> I remember the CAMHS Nurse saying to me over a cup of tea round my kitchen table. Have you ever thought about when you are doing that, what message it sends to your daughter? It really made me stop and think, we talked through some different ideas, and we found a better way forward together, she helped me understand what I needed to do in a supportive, non-judgemental way, that meant a lot and I've not forgotten it.
>
> Parent

Participation with parents and carers needs to be threaded throughout the mental health journey. A care plan loaded with information the family does not understand is almost impossible for a parent to support. If you can help parents understand the 'why' it will make a difference. This might start with helping people understand what terminology means, e.g. CBT (Cognitive Behavioural Therapy), but going even further than this is where the real difference and true partnership between all involved matters.

> I kept being told he has to take positive risks. I had no idea what they meant and was just so scared my son would take his own life I didn't want to leave him for a minute. I slept in his room, I was petrified. I was told I wasn't helping but I didn't know what I should be doing.
>
> Parent

When we start with where parents are and build from there, positive change can happen. What the parent in the quote above needed was somebody to explain what positive risk taking was and the benefits and likely outcomes. Then for this to be introduced in a calm, supportive, staged manner at the child and parents' pace. Unless someone points something out you might not know it is wrong, parents may hear the message differently depending on the emotional state they are in.

For some parents it feels like they can't win. They speak up, ask questions and communicate their support needs to be told they are a 'pushy' or 'savy' parent (both are actual words that have been used to describe parents). They keep quiet, withdraw, or may become defensive or angry when things are suggested and are accused of being a disengaged parent. Behind both is usually a very frightened parent who is doing the best they can to support their child.

> I felt so scared, I was living with the gripping fear I was going to lose my daughter when things were at their worst. I have felt hopeless and a complete failure as a mum. I've felt angry at myself, my daughter, my family and different services along the way. Lost, so many times I was lost for words and what to do.
>
> Parent

The bottom line is, we all want what is best for the child or young person who is struggling with their mental health. If young people, parents, and professionals can work together hand in hand, side by side to try and understand each other's perspective, acknowledging that things can go wrong, and being willing to learn from each other along the way a real difference can be made.

5 Building Resilience

The combination of support, involvement, and increased understanding can build personal resilience which enables parents and carers to feel more confident to cope. There is no better feeling than knowing 'you've got this' or you've had this before, so you will do it again.

Building resilience takes time and everybody's levels of resilience are different depending on a range of other factors that are going on in their lives at the time. The quote 'you never know how strong you are, until being strong is the only choice you have' chimes with so many parents and carers supporting their child with mental health difficulties.

> I have strength I didn't know existed.
>
> Parent

> Before the support group I felt alone, desperate and had no hope. Since attending the group support has been fantastic. I saw that I was not alone and I have gained hope and strength. Without the group I would not be the person I am today.
>
> Parent

Resilience creeps up on you, moment by moment, experience after experience your strength as a parent builds. You learn the language, the system, things that help, things that don't help. You might gain friends and lose friends. You learn about things you never imagined would be part of being a parent. The 'triumph' you feel when you get through a day or night you never thought you could, brings such a relief. When you see your child come through a difficult time it feels so rewarding when you've done something to support them, and it worked.

It is not until you look back, and reflect, that you recognise that as having resilience. On the other hand, when you or someone else has done something that was unintentionally unhelpful, it breaks what can be already very delicate resilience when you are supporting a child with mental health challenges. It's ever changing, it's up and down and experiences that initially appear to break you as a family can end up making you. Because resilience means different things to different people, we will simply explore some of the things that we have learned on our journey and from other parents.

> Just expect, this is life for you now, your daughter will be in and out of inpatient hospitals for the rest of her life.
>
> Professional

Those words from a professional led to one parent who was at a very low point, thinking they would give up. What was the point in still fighting, if this was the life ahead. Words matter, they can knock the fragile confidence of parents and prevent them from reaching out. Thankfully the words from another professional brought balance and helped the parent keep going.

Hold on to hope, that things can get better.

Professional

Hope, like resilience, means different things to different people, but on the dark days when it's hard to see a light at the end of the tunnel-thinking about hope can make you feel stronger. Hope and resilience might look like:

- Knowing there is a 24-hour crisis line if I need it. It can give someone the strength to keep going and get through the night because if the worst happens, they can pick up the phone.
- Trusting your parent instinct and being brave to enough to share thoughts with the professional team. Even better if they are listened to and acted upon.
- Believing I know my child, their likes and dislikes better than the professional team and this knowledge is respected.
- Being included and valued as part of your child's care team.
- Having confidence to speak up and negotiating around what is right for you and your family.
- Feeling less guilty that you are back here after a relapse when things were going so well because you were doing the best you could.
- Daring to put your own oxygen mask on and doing something for yourself when it's the last thing you think you should do.
- Being brave enough to say, I'm stuck, I don't know or I can't do it anymore.
- Saying I wish I wasn't here, but I know what to do and where to reach out to get support.
- Realising you are not alone and finding connections through peer support or experts who cheer you on and encourage you to keep going.
- Asking why? Why are we implementing that, why would that help.
- Having the confidence to speak up and ask for time off at work to support my child because I'm no longer ashamed that my child is struggling.

This list could go on, the most important message we can get across is please ask people what matters to them, what things have helped them in the past, what feels realistic to try. Start from where the family is at. Usually if someone picks the phone up or reaches out, they have exhausted all options available to them at that time. Even if in the past they had managed a similar situation really well, on this occasion they are reaching out. Be curious, ask why, seek to understand. You never know what is going on at this particular moment in time and finding out might help build a picture. In that moment respond to their needs, rather than telling them what you think without really listening. This knowledge will provide needs-led tailored support to the family. So many parents report ringing crisis lines to be told they are not in crisis and encourage their child to do some self-care, e.g. have a bath, paint nails. At this point they are drowning, they need a life ring, not to learn how to swim. That comes later when things are calm.

One parent shared an experience where the mental health team had suggested she sign up to a mindfulness course and was sent information. The parent went along, having arranged for someone to look after her daughter who was experiencing suicidal ideation. Anxiety was high as the parent left the house, to drive to the course, wondering if her daughter was safe. She couldn't concentrate, it was a really difficult hour and she couldn't wait to get home. She didn't want to go back, it felt so stressful but she felt like a failure and she sobbed to a friend who shared an idea that sounded more realistic to her circumstances. It started with one minute of mindfulness with a cup of tea, by the end of the first week the parent was having at least 10 mindful moments a day and it was helping. This was something she could do and of course it helped towards building her resilience.

6 Supporting Others

The whole experience of supporting your child or young person through mental health difficulties often leads to a natural desire for parents to want to support others. The peer support from one parent to another happens when people are given the opportunity to connect. Many parents have set up parent carer support groups in response to there not being one available in their local area. These groups offer a non-judgemental space to share and learn from each other, provide hope, and improve access to services.

> I was able to find out about local services and teams that I can get involved in. Met some people who are going through the same issues we are having or similar. Access to support and info for parents is fab. To be able to speak about your child and not feel like an alien.
>
> Parent

From the seeds of these support groups a new workforce is naturally emerging; parents/carers who have journeyed from navigating support and services for their own children are now providing support to other families. Some have set up independent organisations and others are volunteering or are employed by local Mental Health Trusts or voluntary and community sector organisations. The parent carer peer support workforce is an emerging field, and we are already starting to see the impact of these roles from a parent receiving a service, the parent providing the service, and the professionals who are supporting us.

> Several years ago, my daughter was struggling with his mental health the impact on our family was huge. I felt lost, alone and totally out of my depth. I had to give up work as she was unable to access school, I lost me. I joined a support group and started volunteering to help – it was a lifeline. Fast forward to now- my daughter is in a much better place; family life is back again. I work as a Parent Peer Supporter, and I cannot begin to describe how proud I am to be helping and supporting families who are struggling just like I had. I've come full circle from needing support to supporting others and along the way I found me again.
>
> Parent peer supporter

> You don't know the system or who to turn to. You speak to professionals and you don't understand their language. The professionals know the academic side but they don't feel the total exhaustion and emotion looking after your amazing children. Finding a parent peer support group is worth its weight in gold. They understand your emotions and how to navigate your way through the system, who you need to speak too and what to ask for. They also give you that bit hope that things can get better, when you are rock bottom. Life savers no more words to describe the value of parent peer support.
>
> Parent

> The parent carer peer supporters (PCPS) engage parents in a way statutory service cannot. Parents trust their shared experiences. The PCPS often discover issues with parents that they are unlikely to disclose to services but really block their engagement e.g. literacy problems, previous negative experiences, lack of confidence in working with professionals, feeling unable to speak up and advocate for themselves and their children. PPS often work with complex families as they are the place families go to when they are at their most desperate. PPS are very often highly skilled people with a wealth of knowledge about services across the area and how parents can access the help they need.
>
> Community Modern Matron CYPMHS

Parents and carers from around the country, who run parent carer support groups, helped to form the PLACE Parent Network which is hosted by The Charlie Waller Trust (2022). PLACE provides a space for parents and carers with lived experience of supporting a child with mental health issues and professionals with an interest in parent support, to meet monthly to share practice and ideas. PLACE connects existing parent and carer support groups/projects or those with an interest in developing one.

> It is so good to feel part of a community of parent carer group facilitators to learn from each other and learn together and also to work collaboratively.
>
> PLACE member

The PLACE Network played a key role in supporting the development of the first national Parent Carer Peer Support (PCPS) training programme, which was funded by Health Education England and delivered by a partnership between The Charlie Waller Trust, Charlie Waller Institute, and The Cellar Trust. The training programme aims to help ensure the work parents and carers are doing in communities is recognised and PCPS workers are valued partners in the workforce.

It is life changing when you are supporting a child with mental health difficulties. Everyone's journey is different, but many are left with scars and trauma. It has a whole life impact, from breakdown of friendships and family relationships, to struggling with your own mental health, financial difficulties to leaving employment due to their caring responsibilities. Some are living with every parent's worst fear because their child devastatingly died by suicide, yet many still want to give back to help others through some of the difficulties they experienced.

The parent peer support workforce is one that has foundations in hope. To turn your heartache and difficult life experiences into hope for others is healing. To learn new skills, to contribute to the CYPMH workforce is an honour because we know how much this is needed. It's not easy, demand is high, but you don't want to let anyone down because you know how hard it feels. PCPS workers are at risk of burning out if the right support and infrastructure isn't around them. Professional CYPMH services can work in partnership with parents and carers to help provide a safe, effective service where PCPS workers are offered supervision and clinical advice. This new emerging workforce needs encouragement, support, and understanding – parents and carers are assets and one of the most underused resources in CYPMH, if you work together, it will make a difference to children, young people, families, and professionals' lives.

Ending on a motto that was developed by one of the parent support groups **"We get strong together and do the best we can"** because it applies to each and every one of us.

Top tips for engaging with parents and carers

1   Take the time to build trust and relationships – keep your word and avoid making promises you can't keep.

2 Listen and involve people in the process, talk through what is or is not happening and why.

3 Share tips and strategies used with young people with their parents to help them understand and help their child.

4 Let parents know when their input and ideas have made a difference.

5 Be open to different ideas and be willing to give them a go. This might mean working outside your comfort zone – but it will be worth it.

6 Provide a 'menu' of choice and ways to access support or participation.

7 Offer support, encouragement and try to understand everyone's perspective.

8 Offer practical help, information, training to enable and empower parents.

9 Be honest – if you can't help or implement something – explain why – help parents/young people understand – signpost other ways forward.

10 If you are using digital platforms – keep your camera on, use the chat box or other tools to encourage interaction (if you wouldn't do it face to face don't do it by digital means).

11 If parents are finding it hard to engage – don't give up – ask yourself 'Why?' There is always a way – Ask parents how they want to engage.

12 Don't underestimate the power of a shared cuppa and biscuit – the little things matter.

References

Rollercoaster family support: Mental health support: County Durham (2022). *Rollercoaster Family.* Available at: https://www.rollercoasterfamilysupport.co.uk/ (Accessed: 19 November 2022).

The Charlie Waller Trust (2022). Place - parent support network: Charlie Waller, PLACE - Parent Support Network | Charlie Waller. Available at: https://charliewaller.org/place-parent-support/ (Accessed: 19 November 2022).

Chapter 8

Involving Children, Young People, Parents, and Carers in Service Development

Hannah Sharp (She/Her) and Demi (She/Her)

Introduction: Defining Service Development

It is important to highlight at the start of this chapter that it is not going to discuss participation in relation to 'new service development'. This is where services are developed from scratch. What I shall term 'continuous service development' (CSD), on the other hand, is focused on continuous improvement of existing services and this shall be the focus.

Participation with people with lived experience in new service development is critical, but new service development itself is less common in mental health settings. While there have been emerging examples of new systems of support in recent years, for example via the introduction of Mental Health Support Teams in schools in the UK, the development of a completely new service is something we rarely see, often services are adapted, go through transformation, or are built upon. The principles and discussions around participation throughout this book should be adequate to guide a team through the participation of children and young people, and parent/carers in developing a new service. The principles discussed in this chapter in relation to CSD can also be used as important guidance. The most important consideration within participation in new service development is that it is true participation, with participants involved from the very start, or even before via identification of an area of development.

But what is CSD? To situate CSD in the dialogue surrounding service improvement, it is helpful to first discuss both continuous improvement and quality improvement. Continuous improvement (CI) is about a service continually looking to improve (Bessant et al., 1994), whereas quality improvement (QI) can be an individual or series of projects where the process completes once the desired outcomes are reached (Ovretveit, 2002). These are the most common concepts talked about when discussing how services can improve. CI is inclusive of QI, but a QI initiative is only an aspect of CI. Other aspects of CI include areas such as performance monitoring to allow for the identification of areas where QI

DOI: 10.4324/9781003288800-8

projects can take place – CI looks across the whole service and is more of a principle for how a service ought to conduct itself and its culture, rather than a methodology. I propose that CSD is closest to CI but focuses on the level of the service as a whole. An individual practitioner could seek to continuously improve their own practice, but CSD would be about continually improving whole service practice. CSD is what this chapter focuses on. This is an important distinction to make when it comes to participation, as CSD takes place at the meso- or macro-level (see Chapter 2 for a greater exploration of the 'levels of participation') whereas CI can also take place at the micro-level.

My Experiences Working in Service Development

I have worked across a variety of continuous service development projects over the past nine years in a variety of roles, including as someone with lived experiences and in various roles that did require lived experience, and below I will be anonymously highlighting some of the lessons I have learned from working with services. I will begin with discussion of the challenges I have observed.

The first key challenge I have seen is identifying and reaching out to potential Children and Young People (CYP) and parents/carers to be involved in CSD. Naturally, participation can't occur without a diverse and representative group of people. Often services have felt they do not know how to 'find' and encourage CYP and parent/carers to be involved in participation. Chapter 11 explores how we engage with diverse communities in more detail and the challenges relating to that. But another aspect of this challenge is actually having the capability to find anyone to be involved in participation, regardless of any protected characteristics they may have. Services don't always hold the most up-to-date contact details for past service users or parent/carers, and this can be a critical group to engage with as part of engagement work. Retrospective feedback, once a young person is out of the environment of a service, can often be different once there is time for them to reflect and understand their experiences. For example, for many young people, they are in inpatient settings due to thoughts of ending their life (Mental Health Act, 1983). They do not want to be kept safe for this reason. They may resent staff for trying to keep them safe via restrictive interventions such as restraint or the removal of leave from the unit. However, once they have recovered enough to leave the service, they are more likely, in my experience, to understand why these things happened to them. This often leaves them with a more positive and rounded view of their service. Therefore, in order to get an accurate picture of feedback on the service, retrospective feedback is a critical form of participation and perhaps not always drawn upon. Barriers to this certainly exist, such as CYP not being local to the area, but with the growth of online technology perhaps now is the time to explore this means to work together with past service-users to do CSD. Similar challenges face community services where, in my experience, some CYP don't want to be there either.

The second challenge to discuss is the nature of mental health as ever-changing. Recovery is non-linear (American Psychological Association, 2012) and outcomes and risk, however grounded in evidence-based practice they may be, are uncertain (Dixon and Oyebode, 2007). Naturally, their own mental health impacts on their ability and willingness to participate. The same here goes for parents/carers. Their willingness and ability to participate also may fluctuate based on their young person's current mental state or their own (see Chapter 7 for a model on needing to feel supported before participating). We must adapt how we do participation to reflect this.

In my experience, often services will have one or two young people and parents/carers who are relied on to participate. They are often those who are more naturally vocal about their/their child's care. There are two key problems with this natural reliance. When a CYP or parent/carer is unable to participate for whatever reasons, someone else may not be found and therefore participation does not occur and where participation does occur it is not representative of the wider patient/carer group as it is not possible for one person to represent everyone. Services must consciously engage with and explore means to reach out to other CYP and parents/carers too and ensure this natural reliance does not occur. This will help to mitigate the impact of uncertainty on their ability to engage in participation. Services must also be willing to adapt how they engage with CYP and parents/carers to take account of their current mental state. For example, on a challenging day sitting on an interview panel may be too overwhelming, but helping staff think of interview questions may be manageable. It can sometimes be seen as easier to engage CYP who are further on their recovery journey, but this does not mean others should not be given the opportunity and supported to do so if they wish to participate.

Another challenge I have observed as part of my work is the impact of staffing challenges on participation.

In my experience participation is often driven by a passionate member of staff. If this member of staff leaves, there is no longer someone driving knowledge and motivation to improve participation and go forward. Regardless of whether the member of staff is responsible for participation, passionate or not, if they are to leave then who is to lead the participation work? This requires handover and creates inconsistency, which is problematic when trying to work on an ongoing project. It also requires CYP and parent/carers to build new relationships with a new member of staff – which could be particularly difficult for certain patients (Gunderson,

2007). If participation was embedded, a part of culture and routine, it should be the case that if the lead leaves, the work continues. If the lead leaves and the work stops, this is very telling in itself.

Participation is also often the first thing to 'go' when staffing pressures and competing priorities become too much. For example, in a CYP inpatient unit, if a participation activity is allocated to a member of staff on a particular day, but the staff aren't available, that member of staff may be drafted to other critical duties within the service which have a greater need due to the management of risk. For example, a nurse may be set to lead a community meeting on a unit but due to a member of staff calling in sick they may have to conduct patient observations instead or cover a colleague's appointments for the day. Where services do not have enough staff to account for issues such as illness, as staff shortages would suggest (Ford, 2022), participation falls off the wagon.

This is where a strong, embedded culture of participation is important. Viewing participation as an 'all the time' activity – where the culture of participation is strong it shouldn't have to fall down to a singular member of staff or be scheduled – can help with this. For example, my experience, poor attendance at CYP community inpatient unit meetings is a common challenge. Such meetings are used to gather feedback on the service and so struggling to run these properly is a key missed opportunity for participation. But there are other opportunities to gather feedback to the same level of detail. Why can't these discussions occur from staff having casual chats with patients while they are conducting observations too? Or at the end of an update call with a parent? Or in the community, at the end of a session? Granted, this doesn't have the same dialogue between patients, but there are occasions where this can be achieved, such as at mealtimes or by catching young people at times when they are in a group. Perhaps services need to consider how they record patient and carer feedback and adapt it to allow for these casual occasions of participation.

Continuing on the topic of culture, a positive culture towards participation becomes difficult to maintain with high staff turnover. Organisational culture is founded on shared ideas and attitudes (see Chapter 15). When a cohort changes, these ideas and attitudes are influenced by new people and their own individual ideas and attitudes, as well as being influenced by the absence of the ideas and attitudes from those who have departed the cohort. It takes time for the ideas and attitudes of new staff members to fall into line with those of the existing staff cohort. The higher the level of staff turnover, the more disruption organisational culture faces and the longer it takes for all staff to become aligned.

For more detail on creating culture change within a service, and the way this must be systemic, see Chapter 15.

Having said all this, I wish to emphasise that having a named member of staff responsible for participation isn't a bad thing, and structured occasions of participation are important. But it must come alongside a whole-service responsibility for participation. These casual occasions of participation are often not thought about, but it's important that they are considered as valuable and feedback from them is taken seriously. It is also important to be adaptable to your current patient cohort and the way they want to engage. For some patient cohorts, they could be well-engaged with community meetings and the structure they provide, whereas others may not see the point in them but still express strong opinions about the service day-to-day. Both are equally important means of participation.

The benefits of participation in CSD include all the benefits for services themselves as discussed in Chapter 5. There are two areas of benefits I wish to discuss in more detail here and these are the implementation of more targeted changes, and more meaningful changes.

More targeted changes are those that are able to tackle key issues effectively. Exploring issues with CYP and parents/carers enables services to find the root cause of a problem rather than 'guessing' where it might come from. It also allows a service to work collaboratively to find a solution most likely to make the improvements and have an impact. Meaningful changes on the other hand, are those that matter to the young people and parent/carers the most. If we are focusing on providing person-centred care (as we established in Chapter 6 as crucial to providing effective care), then services need to adapt to meet the needs and wants and likes and dislikes of current patients and parents/carers. These two areas not only result in less wasted resources – including time – but also create more significant improvements in quality as rated by service users and parent/carers as there are improvements in ways that are most impactful for and important to them.

An Expert-by-Experience's Perspective – Demi (She/her)

'**Participation helped secure my future**', is quite a bold statement, but I think it's accurate in a few different ways. Participation helped secure my future, by giving me a purpose at the time, by giving me a role in society again when I couldn't function in education or work, full time. Participation helped secure my future, by giving me things to add to my CV and draw experience to use in interviews, which might otherwise have been a void that I had to explain. Participation helped secure my future, by reshaping a negative experience into a positive one, of learning and growth and informing change.

My experience of mental ill health peaked around 2012–2014, spending time in an inpatient facility and struggling to complete my GCSEs. I had a lot of interaction with the recently formed CAMHS crisis team in the area and was fortunate enough to have my mam be very supportive and engaged with the team, who helped support her to support me. I was one of the first to pilot having a person-centred crisis plan, a plan with decisions made while I was well to support me when I was not, this was one of the things that led to participation as the crisis plan was a success and the team wanted to share their good practice with others.

My participation began by being part of an interview panel for a new crisis team member, alongside my mam and two members of the crisis team, we had a panel of half professional and half lived experience. The interview was for a new member of staff for the crisis team, so it felt important to have the views of people who they'd be working with – others in the team, parents, and young people. The panel, to me, felt truly collaborative, the team had written some questions, and I got to write my own. We all sat together and took it in turns to ask, I was supported on the day with conversations around which questions I felt able to ask and we made the final decision together as a team. I was an equal member, and my scoring was used in the decisions to select the candidate.

When the crisis team were sharing their good practice with others, there was the opportunity for them to present as part of nominations for awards. The team could have presented their work alone, but instead I was able to go along and present from my perspective also, as part of the team. This gave me confidence and presentation skills, which I would otherwise not have had the opportunity to gain. In 2015 we presented for the Nursing Times Awards, the team went on to win the Nursing Times Award for child and adolescent mental health services and were shortlisted for a Patient Safety Award.

The unique part was that the team also invited us to the awards nights – which was unheard of at the time! Participation and lived experience workforce are now becoming part of the vocabulary, but the people we were sharing the table with on the night didn't seem impressed at all (until they wanted a picture with our award!).

Spending the time, outside of crisis, with the team allowed us to build a relationship that enhanced my care and prompted an autism assessment as they'd spent more time with me than an appointment slot. Without that, I don't think I'd have the understanding of myself I now have today.

Reflecting now, 10 years on since the worst part of my mental health, 7 years since the participation work and 6 years since beginning work in a career I love, with no further inpatient stays or intervention needed. I have continued my work in mental health through working behind the scenes with a parent carer support group. I can see the value participation had on my recovery and the impact it has had on my life since. I can now reflect that each part of my journey was for a reason and a team that took a chance on us, broke the mould, and likely made their jobs more complicated as a result, were paving the way for participation without appreciating the profound affect their role would play. Participation secured my future.

Discussion

What Demi's story highlights is how beneficial involvement in CSD can be for service users. Similar benefits also extend to parents and carers. Demi's experience as one of the trailblazers of participation shows that new initiatives can and do work. Teams shouldn't be afraid to try out new things relating to participation. When done well, even if it doesn't contribute to huge service change, it can be life-changing for a young person and even therapeutic.

Conclusion

To summarise the key takeaways from this chapter; service must be conscious of involving the right people in participation. They must ensure it is a diverse group, including those who have left the service. This comes with challenges, and services must be set-up to overcome these. Despite these challenges, participation in CSD has significant benefits for both the service and service users. With the right level of thought and preparation, participation works.

References

American Psychological Association, 2012. Recovery principles. *American Psychological Association* 43, 55.

Bessant, J., Caffyn, S., Gilbert, J., Harding, R., Webb, S., 1994. Rediscovering continuous improvement. *Technovation* 14, 17–29. https://doi.org/10.1016/0166-4972(94)90067–90061.

Dixon, M., Oyebode, F., 2007. Uncertainty and risk assessment. *Advances in Psychiatric Treatment* 13, 70–78. https://doi.org/10.1192/apt.bp.105.002022.

Ford, M., 2022. Nurse vacancies across England remain "stubbornly high". *Nursing Times.* https://www.nursingtimes.net/news/workforce/nurse-vacancies-across-england-remain-stubbornly-high-04-03-2022/ (accessed 11. 4. 2022).

Gunderson, J. G., 2007. Disturbed relationships as a phenotype for borderline personality disorder. *AJP* 164, 1637–1640. https://doi.org/10.1176/appi.ajp.2007.07071125.

Mental Health Act, 1983. Statute Law Database.

Ovretveit, J., 2002. Evaluation of quality improvement programmes. *Quality and Safety in Health Care* 11, 270–275. https://doi.org/10.1136/qhc.11.3.270.

Chapter 9

Involving Children and Young People in Mental Health Research

Cathy Street (She/Her) and Amanda Cooper (She/Her)

Introduction

This chapter explores how children and young people (CYP) with lived experience of Children and Young People's Mental Health (CYPMH) services can be involved in mental health research. Drawing on the lived experience of one of the authors, it explains the key role CYP can play through their involvement in small, local studies of, for example, a specific mental health service or new intervention, through to large-scale international studies, which might involve piloting a major service improvement initiative, a randomised controlled trial (RCT) or a longitudinal study.

CYP can be involved in many different ways. This depends on what is appropriate for their age and stage of development, as well as the nature, duration, and location of the research study. It is equally important to consider the child or young person's interests, including their existing expertise or the skills they might wish to acquire. The capacity of the research team to provide any training that might be needed, as well as support throughout to the CYP, and possibly for young children, parents, or carers, must also be considered.

CYP are often key subjects of, and participants in, mental health research. This may be via interviews, focus groups, surveys and increasingly, the use of creative approaches such as the use of film, drama, music and art (Street et al. 2016; Leigh 2020). The advantages of the latter are now widely recognised in terms of both engagement with CYP and gathering insightful data. For example, Dunn and Mellor (2017) highlight that participatory, collaborative research can be especially engaging for vulnerable or seldom heard voices and that creative approaches can help young people to share sensitive topics in innovative ways.

This theme is echoed by McLaughlin (2015) who mentions the work of Roberts (2004) who argues that involving children in research is not only effective, it promotes democratic and active citizenship. It also allows adult researchers greater awareness of children's worlds, and this is important: "just because we have all been children we cannot assume we understand the

DOI: 10.4324/9781003288800-9

world of the children of today" (McLaughlin 2015: 14). This is pointed out by a young person involved in a large international mental health study:

> Involving those who use services is the only way services can truly reflect current wants and needs. Involving young people in research is an important part of this and really connects up research and reality. The voice of lived experience is very powerful.
>
> Young person

In terms of having a direct research role, as opposed to being a participant or research subject from whom data is being sought, CYP can: act as advisors to a study, including at the grant application stage; sit on a study's steering group; work as peer researchers helping to design and pilot the research tools (e.g., questionnaires and interview schedules); support the research team to engage with and retain study participants; undertake interviews or run focus groups, either on their own or as co-facilitators. Later on, they may be involved in the analysis of data, writing up of reports and the dissemination of findings.

In this chapter, the focus is the benefits and the challenges of involving CYP with lived experience as part of a research team. Much of this material draws on real-life research studies that the authors have been directly involved in over the last 10–15 years. We consider what needs to be in place to make children and young people's (CYPs) involvement safe, ethical, and meaningful to young people themselves – what might be called 'good practice' in the research field. Our conclusions summarise some of the challenges for the future and make recommendations for how these might be addressed.

The National Policy Context

At an over-arching level, the United Nations Convention on the Rights of the Child (1989) is an important influence on CYPs involvement in all areas of service provision that affect them, with Article 12 in particular setting out their right to say what they think and to have their views taken seriously (Dunn and Mellor 2017). Such a stance underpins key documents such as Future in Mind (Department of Health and NHS England 2015) where the participation and involvement of CYP in CYPMH services is a central theme.

Turning specifically to mental health research, national policy is strongly supportive of CYPs involvement, recognising that this brings a wide range of benefits. Indeed, some funders, including the National Institute for Health and Care Research (NIHR), require evidence of Patient and Public Involvement (PPI) as part of considering a research grant application, describing public involvement as a core principle in the way it works (Jenner et al. 2015).

Furthermore, INVOLVE, an NIHR-funded body, states that CYP should be offered a choice and flexibility of involvement options from early on in the research process and that this must not be tokenistic (Kirby 2004).

In its guide UK Standards for Public Involvement (INVOLVE 2019), six key areas are set out, namely that there should be:

- Inclusive opportunities
- Working together that values all contributions
- Support and learning opportunities
- Communications that are well-timed and relevant
- Impact that is identified and shares the difference that public involvement made
- Governance that supports the involvement of the public in research management, leadership and decision-making.

More recently, the NHS Health Research Authority (HRA) published a briefing "Putting people first – embedding public involvement in health and social care" (HRA 2022). Applying to all ages, this states in the introduction that:

> Public involvement is important, expected, and possible in all types of health and social care research ... People have the right to be involved in all health and social care research. Excellent public involvement is an essential part of health and social care research and has been shown to improve its quality and impact. People's lived experiences should be a key driver...

Ethical Requirements

Ethical considerations are a key part of the mental health research landscape, not least since studies typically concern sensitive and often highly personal issues that may be profoundly affecting those under study. Most studies, in the UK and also internationally, are required to seek ethical approval from a Research Ethics Committee (REC) before any direct data gathering can commence. In setting out a study's proposed methodology, this should detail the proposed role of all researchers in the team, including any CYP members recruited for their lived-experience expertise.

According to INVOLVE, since 2010, the HRA and INVOLVE have, on a biennial basis, analysed the extent of public involvement in REC applications; they explain that the information provided by researchers about this can provide assurances and greatly assist the ethical review. INVOLVE has reported that the HRA was reviewing how it could put greater emphasis on assessing public involvement as part of ethical review

(INVOLVE and NHS Health Research Authority 2016), with the Nuffield Council on Bioethics (2015) noting:

> Research ethics committees (RECs) should routinely require researchers to have involved children, young people and parents, as appropriate, in the design of their studies. Researchers who have not sought input in this way should be required to justify to the research ethics committee why this was not appropriate in their case.
>
> (Nuffield Council on Bioethics 2015, p.xxvii)

The Multi-faceted Benefits of Involving Children and Young People

The benefits of involving CYP in CYPMH are multi-faceted and can bring both immediate and longer-term impacts for three, quite distinct, groups: firstly, those with lived experience, secondly, research participants and thirdly, researchers and those working in the policy world who draw on research evidence in developing new, or updating existing, health policy and guidance.

For CYP with Lived Experience

Giving CYP a **'voice' or direct representation** is possibly one of the most important benefits. Voicing opinions on the mental healthcare CYP receive can be both empowering and cathartic for the CYP involved. It can provide an in-depth snapshot of the current situation of services, drawing on the CYPs unique experiences of mental health disorders and the care offered, good or otherwise. Such perspectives can shed light on the more subtle ways in which professional agendas may dominate; whether and how services feel welcoming to CYP (or not); whether information is well communicated and decisions are mutually agreed (or not), and the extent to which the issues of concern to the young person feel acknowledged (or not).

Recognition of lived experience expertise supports an approach wherein research is done 'with' or 'by', rather than 'to', 'about' or 'for' CYP, which implies both a much more passive role for CYP and the dominance of professional viewpoints. Telling their story can allow CYP to reflect on their experiences and the experiences of others in similar situations: "reframing negative past experiences as learning to drive positive change can be empowering and satisfying" (CFE Research 2020, p.3).

They can distinguish between policy, policy into practice and how the two can vary through many different factors, insights that can be highly useful in national service transformation initiatives and identification of areas for future research.

Participation in research can aid **recovery and wellbeing**. This could be through reflection on own experiences; increased knowledge about mental health; the validation of experiences and the promotion of hope, as one young person involved in the MILESTONE pan-European study (Tuomainen et al. 2018) noted: "it showed me I am more than my diagnosis... It helped me in my personal recovery".

Feelings of isolation adversely affect many CYP with mental health problems and involvement in research **can help CYP feel less alone, assist them to explain their health difficulties to others, both peers and health professionals.** These and other benefits are identified in recent research using mixed methods that explored the usefulness of developing and sharing a suite of lived experience research resources that covered topics such as 'what helps recovery' and 'getting physical health care' (Honey et al. 2020).

Furthermore, many CYP who have experience of CYPMH services want to 'give something back to others', which may be in terms of sharing what worked or alternatively, highlighting practice or mental health provision that needs to be improved. As one young person involved in research about transition from CYPMH services commented: "I wanted to take my bad experience and use it in the hope of helping other young people".

Involvement in research can provide CYP with **learning opportunities and the acquisition of transferable skills,** which are highly useful in terms of potentially improving future employment opportunities; they can also gain self-confidence and self-esteem (Shaw et al. 2011). Apart from research skills (e.g., interviewing, data analysis and report writing) and knowledge about mental health, CYP can learn about new technology, for example app-building or film-making.

CYP may also acquire presentation and public-speaking expertise, knowledge of different cultures or national and local government policies; skills in appraisal and reflection, peer support, multi-agency and team working. For some CYP, their engagement in research can **build and foster confidence in daily living skills,** such as travelling on public transport and the planning, scheduling and reporting of activities to others.

For Research Participants

Research by INVOLVE and NHS Health Research Authority (2016) concluded that PPI supports a more respectful and ethically acceptable use of people's time and plays a crucial role in the process of consent, notably it can help improve participant information sheets (HRA 2022), with poor information materials often being a cause for RECs not giving approval. They suggest that PPI in designing the consent process makes it more likely that **consent will be genuinely 'informed'** by ensuring that potential research participants receive the information they want and need, delivered in clear and accessible ways, which reflect their interests and concerns. Furthermore, PPI can positively shape the entire consent process, by identifying the most appropriate times to invite people to join a study, the frequency of contact with researchers and the best times to collect data that may be sensitive or distressing.

The HRA suggests that involvement of those with lived experience **can aid research with people from diverse cultural backgrounds**. Involving people from different communities and promoting inclusivity can facilitate awareness of any ethical concerns that may be specific to a particular community (HRA 2022). The involvement of people with lived experience as peer researchers can put them in a stronger position to be able to empathise with participants and to validate experiences that are reported.

Other research suggests that the **actual experience of participating in research may be improved**. It has been reported that PPI in research design is likely to ensure that practical arrangements required by participants are addressed and any burden is minimised – for example, the selection of convenient local venues for interviews and the reimbursement of expenses (Jenner et al. 2015; Staley 2015). PPI can also help ensure that both the length and frequency of any assessments or interviews are appropriate.

For the Research World

Possibly the most important benefit to researchers is that the involvement of CYP with lived experience is that this can **'ground' research and helps to ensure that it is picking up on real-life concerns**, not just what academics, politicians or research funders may be interested in. It can improve focus, help prioritisation of the key areas to be studied and can promote a sense of credibility, that there is an evidenced reason to do the research. Involvement can provide a challenge to researcher thinking, planning, values and communication, "a process that researchers describe as a 'a lightbulb moment' or 'reality check'" (Staley 2015: 7).

In their analysis of the role of lived experience experts in systems change, CFE notes: "Experts provide a powerful and authentic voice and unique insights that can challenge assumptions, motivate organisations to do things differently and pinpoint areas for change" (CFE Research 2020: 3). From the perspective of mental health research, this is highly relevant since often what sits behind a mental health research study is the wish to address some area of concern about professional practice or CYPMH service provision.

A variety of research studies about the involvement of people with lived experience also propose that this can help to **challenge stigmatising perspectives and stereotypes**, in this case, with regard to CYP with mental health difficulties. For example, there may be views that due to either

CYPs age and/or illness, their opinions may be unreliable. Alternatively, some may hold the view that it is inappropriate to involve CYP for fear of aggravating their mental health difficulties, triggering a deterioration in their mental state.

Of course, this is possible but, perhaps more pertinently, this latter concern points to the importance of research that is undertaken in ways that are safe, planned with advice, guidance and support embedded. A further benefit, according to CFE is that involvement of people with lived experience has the potential to reduce power imbalances (CFE Research 2020).

The involvement of those with lived experience **can improve actual research activities and outputs**, leading to better data quality from potentially more representative and diverse audiences. Honey and colleagues (2020) suggest that it can enhance methodological sensitivity and improve data accuracy, validity and results, which in turn can help make the findings seem more relevant to service users. Similar points are made in "Putting people first" (HRA 2022). Some of the specific benefits identified include:

- Improved recruitment of research participants (Ennis and Wykes 2013; Crocker et al. 2018)
- Where peer researchers are involved, participants are more likely to be honest about their experiences (CFE Research 2020)
- More informed analysis, drawing on service user insights (Russell et al. 2020); PPI has been found to promote richness of data, possibly by supporting different, more experiential approaches to coding data (Jennings et al. 2018)
- Accessible findings providing wider and more relevant viewpoints and dissemination via 'user-friendly' ways; these give better credibility with stakeholders (Sales et al. 2021) and better overall reach to those who use, provide, or plan and commission, health services.

In summary, the involvement of people with lived experience brings a wide range of different benefits for different groups: it can be empowering of CYP providing news skills and validation of their experiences; it can support the engagement of diverse groups; it can 'ground' research, and it can lead to clear improvements in the quality, robustness and relevance of research activities and the data produced.

Does CYPs Involvement Really Work?

Some researchers have challenged the assumed benefits of public involvement or co-production with people with lived experience in health research. For example, some have talked of a tendency to present involvement as a right and therefore of value irrespective of any impact (Staley 2015). However, many do not agree with this, and recent years have seen an emphasis on developing the evidence base for PPI and ways to demonstrate its impact, including via systematic reviews, realist evaluations, studies of stakeholder views and the development of frameworks and guidance (Russell et al. 2020; Jenner et al. 2015).

There have also been questions as to whether the costs outweigh the benefits, what Oliver and colleagues (2019) call "the dark side of coproduction". Others have raised concerns that much of the evidence is weak and anecdotal (Staley 2015); that any negative impacts are rarely discussed (Russell et al. 2020), and that the impact of CYPs involvement in research is an understudied area (Sales et al. 2021).

Oliver et al. (2019) suggest that there is little consensus about co-production, including what it actually entails, the reasons for it and the best techniques to use and with whom. They go on to explain that it is not risk or cost free (to those with lived experience, researchers, and wider stakeholder groups) and that there can be tensions between the different interests involved. Rather than generating rich and insightful data that draws on lived experiences, they warn that the co-production process in research can lead to findings that are not generalizable since they can be overly focused on local issues – and therefore, not easily publishable either. They conclude that whilst there are many promising examples, there remain many unanswered questions and a more reflective and open discussion is needed about how the research process, and the different roles and responsibilities of everyone involved, may be affected.

Staley's (2015) exploration of how to measure the impact of PPI in research draws similar conclusions. This work highlights that much PPI is highly context dependent and can take many different forms, encompassing multiple activities at different levels, for example, strategic and operational, local, and national.

In terms of the negative impacts of involving people with lived experience, some studies suggest that for those who get involved, there can be feelings of overwork, frustration, and marginalisation if there is limited opportunity to influence the direction of the research. There can also be conflict and confusion about the PPI role, time, and financial burdens (Russell et al. 2020; Jenner et al. 2015).

Russell and colleagues (2020) also caution that whilst well-intentioned, the setting of national standards can have the disadvantage of becoming prescriptive, defining and bounding PPI in a constricting way. It can feed the problem of tokenism in PPI, and rather than being empowering or emancipatory, can have the opposite effect – especially where it feels that researchers are being driven to involve people with lived experience only to satisfy the reporting requirements of funding bodies and ethics committees.

Meaningful Involvement

According to CFE's research, for involvement to be meaningful there is a need for cultural change and a shift in attitudes (CFE Research 2020). Their analysis of the role of lived experience in systems change identifies a number of things that can ensure that CYPs involvement in research is meaningful and not tokenistic and include:

- Buy-in to CYPs involvement across the organisation, with willingness to adapt to make the most of the opportunity
- Avoidance of one-off or 'tick box' activities and ideally, the development of lasting opportunities, such as membership of advisory or strategy boards
- Addressing any power differential between academics and CYP by ensuring full integration of CYP within the team, with mutual respect and opportunities to share opinions which are truly listened to
- Provision of a dedicated contact or co-ordinator for PPI who experts know and trust, also access to emotional support that is tailored and can be varied over time as required, and time with peers for mutual support and sharing of experiences
- Ensuring that experts with lived experience are kept informed throughout and receive timely feedback and debriefing; information provided in advance of meetings allows lived experience experts to prepare, play an active role and not be 'just another item on the agenda'
- Not pressuring or expecting experts with lived experience to share personal experiences unless they wish to do so.

The role of a dedicated PPI co-ordinator or facilitator can greatly influence the success of CYP involvement in research. A named person that bridges the gap between lived experience, the wider research team, and mental health professionals can be pivotal in breaking down any barriers between the different groups, including any confusion about different roles and responsibilities.

A co-ordinator can ensure CYPs voices are heard in large meetings or events and can help those with lived experience to feel able to challenge the use of jargon or unexplained medical terms, which may be particularly prevalent in clinical studies. If travelling locally or internationally, having a point of contact can boost CYPs self-esteem in interpersonal skills such as writing, reading, presenting, and travelling. In the experience of one of the authors, contact between the PPI co-ordinator can also be more relaxed by using texts or WhatsApp messages, rather than formal emails that can sometimes feel quite daunting.

Barriers to CYPs Involvement in Research

A variety of barriers can impede the involvement of CYP with lived experience in research about CYPMH services. Many of these are described in the literature that has explored the impact of patient and public involvement or co-production. For example, the reviews by Staley (2015), Oliver et al. (2019) and Russell et al. (2020) mention, among other things:

- **Time and administrative burden**: research involving those with lived experience may take longer and need more preparation, training, and flexibility in how activities and who is involved (being mindful of the other commitments of those with lived experience) are scheduled; all may be at odds with funder requirements
- **Money and resource needs** are likely to be higher. Oliver et al. (2019) note that doing research in this way is expensive since it requires the presence of multiple actors who often have other primary responsibilities; however, as Russell and colleagues (2020) warn, under resourcing can lead to perceptions of tokenism and negate the value of the involvement of those with lived experience
- **Communication and information sharing** – which can be impaired by REC or local health trust restrictions as to what data can be shared and with whom
- The interpersonal skills needed to **recruit and manage what may be a highly mixed group** working together, skills which not all academics may be trained in or possess (Oliver et al. 2019), and where it is crucial not to allow powerful voices to dominate proceedings
- **Research focus that cannot reflect the values and priorities of all stakeholders**, which may be demotivating for CYP with lived experience to stay involved unless this is well managed in terms of looking for ways to make the study relevant to these groups
- **Ensuring the representativeness and diversity of CYP can also be difficult** to achieve. In many cases, research about CYPMH services involves those currently using services, or with recent use, often due to difficulties contacting those who have disengaged from or been accepted into mainstream services – but who may very well have important experiences to share.

Case Study: The MILESTONE Project

MILESTONE (Tuomainen et al. 2018) was a five-year, pan-European research study about young people's transition from CYPMH services to Adult Mental Health Services (AMHS). Success of the project's PPI included winning the charity MQ Mental Health and National Institute for Health and Care Research (NIHR) Service User Involvement in Research Award in 2016. Reflecting on what sat behind this, the CYP who worked on MILESTONE as young project advisors (YPAs) identified the following:

- They were involved from the very start, had contracts from the host organisation the University of Warwick, with these renewable on an annual basis and setting out agreed, but flexible, hours of work and rates of pay
- A senior member of the research team had dedicated responsibility for PPI, ensuring that the CYP were kept informed of all developments, that opportunities for involvement were shared and that CYPs individual interests and skills, or those they wished to acquire, were considered in planning activities, training, and support
- There was commitment for the YPAs to be fully involved in all aspects of the study as members of the research team: they advised on the research tools in the development stage; attended all steering group meetings in different study partner countries, with a slot allocated for PPI; presented at dissemination events and conferences, contributed to the writing of the final report and articles for journals
- The use of CYP-led creative approaches, which included the making of three short films. One of these drew on a poetry workshop wherein the YPAs and the researchers created a poem and associated imagery for a work titled *I am the Loneliness of 4am*, which is how one of the CYP had experienced their transition from CYPMH services.
- Reflecting on their involvement as a Young Project Advisor in MILESTONE, one of the authors noted it was:

One of the best things I have participated in! It was a once in a lifetime opportunity that I will always be grateful for. To be a part of pivotal research internationally for me, was an honour. I gained so much confidence in public speaking and was able to speak in front of researchers both nationally and internationally. I was able to make friends for life not only in the UK but in different countries with those also wanting to improve mental health provisions in their countries.

- Furthermore:

as young project advisors we were able to recruit and then mentor the next wave of advisors from Ireland. I gained confidence in travelling internationally to the different bi-yearly meetings. I am very passionate to turn my negative experience of being a service user into helping others not to go through the same as I did and I feel mental health research involving CYP is a significant factor in aiding mental health service transformation.

Some of the Barriers Encountered

- MILESTONE was a long project which made keeping CYP involved as advisors difficult as their circumstances, including their mental health, changed. This was addressed by having a flexible approach to who was involved, when and for what activities, with some young people taking 'time out', e.g., for exams, and a snowballing approach to recruiting new YPAs as the project progressed.
- There was a very large team of researchers working across eight different countries administering a wide range of complex assessments at multiple time points; apart from time pressures and language barriers, there were some cultural differences in how PPI was viewed and researcher confidence in co-production with CYP varied; research ethics committee requirements of the different countries also prevented the sharing of some data.
- Having a dedicated PPI lead to support CYP and ensuring that there were always several YPAs involved, flexibly, undoubtedly required a well-funded PPI budget and a considerable time commitment, including for travel, of both CYP and the PPI lead.
- The research was very complex, and one of the co-authors directly experienced, "there was a lot of jargon we had to get our heads round" and the different work packages (quote usual in big studies) could be confusing to follow.

Conclusions

The UK national policy environment is strongly supportive of, and increasingly expects to see, PPI in research. Within this context, our review of the role of CYP with lived experience in research about CYPMH Services highlights a range of clear benefits that come from undertaking research in a participatory and collaborative fashion with CYP, but also a number of important barriers to be considered.

In terms of advantages, we have explained how some distinct groups, namely, those CYP who are involved, research participants, researchers and those working in policy arenas can all benefit. Involvement of CYP can give CYP a 'voice' and recognition of the expertise arising from their lived experience. It can aid their recovery and wellbeing by boosting self-confidence, self-esteem, the promotion of hope and the reduction of feelings of isolation; it can also provide longer-term advantages through offering learning and opportunities to acquire transferable skills.

Where there is a sense of teamwork, co-production can have a genuinely positive effect on research processes and outputs. If CYP feel they are part of a team, are valued and supported they will be more likely to have an active involvement and complete tasks; at a personal level, they are likely to be energised and inspired by each other and can form great, lifelong friendships with like-minded people, undoubtedly of significant value to their mental health and wellbeing and to mental health services overall.

Turning to research participants, benefits include improvements in the process of consent and the addressing of practical arrangements. There can be greater sensitivity to ensuring that research participants are not overly burdened and are supported and informed. For the research and policy world, research literature emphasises how the involvement of those with lived experience can 'ground' research in real life, challenge assumptions and mental health stigma and help to address power imbalances. PPI can also improve specific research activities including the interpretation and analysis of data and the dissemination of findings.

Set against these, some researchers have challenged the lack of evidence as to these claimed benefits and called for robust empirical research; they have also questioned the assumption that public involvement is a right and therefore is automatically of value. This more critical area of the literature identifies some of the potential barriers to involvement; these include higher costs; the need for more time; risks of role confusion and interpersonal conflict. There can be problems with people feeling frustrated or marginalised if their influence on the focus or direction of the research can only be limited, which can also make involvement seem tokenistic or experienced as a 'tick box' activity.

Whilst acknowledging limitations in the evidence base, however, other researchers have drawn attention to the unique way that PPI can have an impact on the whole process of research and cautioned that its effects are more subtle than, for example, just analysing costs and time.

We conclude with some words from a MILESTONE Young Project Advisor which we feel sum up succinctly why involvement of CYP in research about CYPMH services is important and must be embedded in future studies, drawing on the ideas of what 'good practice' in this field summarised earlier in this chapter, might include:

> If participation in research didn't exist, there would be no voice for young people, they would feel marginalised … Being involved in research relies on the willingness to learn and evolve healthcare. But without this motivation, care would become stagnant or even deteriorate. It's imperative to the parity of esteem cause and the stigma surrounding mental health.

References

CFE Research (2020) The role of lived experience in creating systems change. Evaluation of fulfilling love: supporting people with multiple, needswww.cfe.org.uk.

Crocker, J., Ricci-Cabello, I., Servet, M., Parker, A., Hirst, J., Chant, A., Petit-Semain, S., Evans, D., and Rees, S. (2018) Impact of patient and public involvement on enrolment and retention in clinical trials: systematic review and meta-analysis. *BMJ* 363, https://doi.org/10.1136/bmj.k4738.

Department of Health and NHS England (2015) Future in mind – promoting, protecting and improving our children and young people's mental health and wellbeing, https://assets.publishing.service.gov.uk.

Dunn, V. and Mellor, T. (2017) Creative, participatory projects with young people: Reflections over five years. *Research for All* 1(2), 284–299, https://doi.org/10.18546/RFA.01.2.05.

Ennis, L. and Wykes, T. (2013) Impact of patient involvement in mental health research: Longitudinal study. *British Journal of Psychiatry* 203(5), 381–386.

Honey, A., Boydell, K., Coniglio, F., Thuy Do, T., Dunn, L., Gill, K., Glover, H., Hines, M., Newton Scanlon, J. and Tooth, B. (2020) Lived experience research as a resource for recovery: a mixed methods study. *BMC Psychiatry* 20(456) https://doi.org/10.1186/s1288-020-02861-0.

INVOLVE (2019) UK Standards for Public Involvementwww.invo.org.uk.

INVOLVE and NHS Health Research Authority (2016) Impact of public involvement on the ethical aspects of researchwww.invo.org.uk.

Jenner, M., Gilchrist, M. and Baker, G. (2015) Practical considerations in improving research through public involvement Research. *Involvement and Engagement* 1(3) https://doi.org/10.1186/s40900-015-002-y.

Jennings, H., Slade, M., Bates, P., Munday, E. and Toney, R. (2018) Best practice framework for Patient and Public Involvement (PPI) in collaborative data analysis of qualitative mental health research: Methodology development and refinement. *BMC* 18(1), 213, https://doi.org/10.1186/s12888-018-1794-8.

Kirby, P. (2004) *A Guide to Actively Involving Young People in Research: For researchers, research commissioners and managers.* Eastleigh, INVOLVE, www.invo.org.uk.

Leigh, J. (2020) Using creative research methods and movement to encourage reflection in children. *Journal of Early Childhood Research* 18(2), 130–142.

McLaughlin, H. (2015) Ethical issues in the involvement of children and young people in research in McLaughlin, H. (ed) *Involving Children and Young People in Policy, Practice and Research.* London, National Children's Bureau, www.yhscn.nhs.uk.

NHS Health Research Authority (HRA) (2022) Putting people first – embedding public involvement in health and social care research, www.hra.nhs.uk.

Nuffield Council on Bioethics (2015) Children and clinical research: ethical issueswww.nuffieldbioethics.org.

Oliver, K., Kothari, A. and Mays, N. (2019) The dark side of coproduction: do the costs outweigh the benefits for health research? *Health Research Policy and Systems* 17(33) https://doi.org/10.1186/s12961-019-0432-3.

Roberts, H. (2004) Health and Social Care, in Fraser, S. *et al.* (eds) *Doing Research with Children and Young People.* London: Sage.

Russell, J., Fudge, N. and Greenhalgh, T. (2020) The impact of public involvement in health research: what are we measuring? Why are we measuring it? Should we stop measuring it? *Research Involvement and Engagement* 6(63) https://doi.org/10.1186/s40900-020-00239-w.

Sales, C., Martins, F., Alves, M., Carletto, S., Conejo-Ceron, S., Costa da Silva, L. and Edbrooke-Childs, J. (2021) Patient and public involvement in youth mental health research: protocol for a systematic review of practices and impact. *Frontiers in Psychology*, November, 12 https://doi:10.3389/fpsyg.2021.703624.

Shaw, C., Brady, L. and Davey, C. (2011) Guidelines for research with young people. London, National Children's Bureau, www.info.lse.ac.uk.

Staley, K. (2015) 'Is it worth doing?' Measuring the impact of patient and public involvement in research. *Research Involvement and Engagement* 1(6) https://DOI10.1186/s40900-015-0008-5.

Street, C., Wallace, E., Joshi, P. and Williams, L. (2016) Listening to young children in practice: using and adapting the Mosaic approach. *Social Research Practice* 2.

Tuomainen, H., Schulze, U., Warwick, J., Paul, M., Dieleman, G., Franic, T., Madan, J., Maras, A., McNicholas, F., Purper-Ouakil, D., Santosh, P., Signorini, G., Street, C., Tremmery, S., Verhulst, F., Wolke, D. and Singh, S.P. for the MILESTONE Consortium (2018) Managing the link and strengthening transition from child to adult mental health care in Europe (MILESTONE): Background, rationale and methodology. *BMC Psychiatry* 18(167) https://doi.org/10.1186/s12888-018-1758-z.

Chapter 10

Involving Younger Children

Ann Cox (She/Her)

Introduction

This chapter will review how to involve younger children in participation. It will provide an overview of child development and how adaptations will need to be made depending on the developmental stage of the child. This chapter will explore communications methods which can enhance participation for the younger child. Consideration will be given to the potential barriers when involving younger children in participation and how to overcome them. This chapter will include reviewing consent and agreement for participation from the child. It will also explore some challenges that can come with child consent and how to negotiate these with the parent or caregiver.

Why it is Important to Involve Younger Children?

The following quote from the Chinese philosopher Xun Kuang is a helpful reminder about how children learn best:

> Tell me and I forget, teach me and I may remember, involve me and I learn.
>
> (312–230 BC)

Involving children in participation has many benefits for the child. Children who are involved in decision-making activities will be developing and improving their cognitive skills and function. This will further improve the child's decision-making abilities and in their adult lives (Cox, 2021). Children who are involved in such activities further have improved self-esteem, self-agency, and motivation (Ruddock & McIntyre, 2007; Cox et al., 2010; Davies et al., 2005; Hannam, 2001). Being involved in participation can also improve children's social inclusion and their capacity and competence in decision-making activities. This highlights the benefits for involving younger children, increasing the potential for improved

DOI: 10.4324/9781003288800-10

personal and cognitive development (Brooker and Woodhead, 2008; Larcher and Hutchinson, 2010).

Child Development and How this Impacts on Involving Children in Participation

Child development is measured by the physical and cognitive maturation of the child. Child development has been theorised in many different ways. Piaget (1964) theorised that child development is chronological and directly aligned to the age of the child, and Erikson (1980) theorised that there are eight stages to child development based on psychosocial development. Bronfenbrenner (1979) suggests that child development is based on ecological, systemic change, whilst Klaczynski (2004) theorises that there is a dual processing theory to child development. This includes a chronological maturation alongside an experiential or heuristic development. There has not been an agreed theory that fully explains the complexities of child development, however using a collective view of these theories includes a range of possible influences to child development. What we do know is that children develop individually, for example, two seven year olds will never be in exactly the same development stage. They might have similarities such as be at the same reading level, but their comprehension, physical development and abstract thinking skills are likely to be different. Therefore, caution should always be taken when working with a group of children the same age and expecting their understanding, competence or ability to participate to be the same.

Many factors positively and negatively influence child development. From a positive perspective, it is well known that children who are brought up in loving and nurturing environments are more likely to develop well and align to the optimal developmental norms (Tan and Fegert, 2004; Maslow, 1943). Children who are provided a wide range of activities to engage in, have outdoor play, and explore the world during childhood will also thrive (Moss, 2012). For a child to be able to engage in a positive childhood, these factors also have to align to the optimal physical health of the child. Any physical illness, learning disability, or injury may hinder or reduce the ability of a child to develop to their fullest.

It is always helpful to consider the child's stage of development, rather than base understanding on the chronological age of the child. Assessing the developmental stage of child can be difficult, however, understanding how the child may be most receptive to information will be important to ensure that the child has the best opportunity to engage in participation. Younger children tend to enjoy more visual and 'hands on' ways of engaging. This is because younger children will not have developed their full processing abilities as yet, so seeing things visually can be a better way to engage them. This may be in the form of pictures, questionnaires, drawings, using pens, pencils, toys, paper or white boards (Cox, 2021). Older children may have the ability, depending on the stage of their development, to think more abstractly and mentalise concepts better than what younger children can do. Mentalising is being able to conceptualise an idea in the imagination (Peterson, 2022). It is a form of processing, where the verbal or written information is conceptualised as an idea in the imagination. An example of this could be if it were asked of someone to give you directions from their home to their local supermarket, they would be able to conceptualise that idea in their head, picture the roads and route they would have to take to get to the local supermarket. This ability to mentalise is something children develop throughout childhood and therefore is a skill that is honed during cognitive maturation. A younger child may struggle to do this, so you would need to help them understand concepts in a more visual way, rather than asking them to process cognitively.

An important aspect to Lindahal et al.'s (2004) child development theory was the concept of heuristics and how children learn. Klaczynski (*ibid*) agreed with Piaget (1964) and other theories that there was a maturation of the child through physical and cognitive development, however they also theorised that children further develop through experience and heuristics. This involves each individual experience of the child. The child stores each experience or memory of these events. When a child finds themselves in a similar experience later in life, then the child will automatically and at times unconsciously draw on these memories to inform their response to the situation in front of them. Therefore, by children experiencing many situations they will develop an increasing repository of heuristics to draw on and in doing so will have the ability to make better choices in situations in the future. When involving children in participation and by helping them engage in new situations or experiences, the children will be developing new heuristics. This will help them in the future to become better decision-makers and more confident in their abilities. It is really important that all professionals help children engage in new experiences which support the development of new heuristics, which in turn will improve their future decision-making abilities.

Impact of Mental Health Difficulties

Mental health difficulties can hinder the development of the child. The mental health of a child can impact cognitive functioning and reasoning, reducing the child's ability to process situations, manage strong and distressing emotions and manage social and domestic relationship dynamics. For example, a child with anxiety may struggle to think in class because they have so many worries that they are thinking about, and therefore the child does not have the headspace to process what is being taught in class. As a result, their ability to take in and comprehend information will be reduced. The child then may not want to go to school due to feeling inadequate or that it is too much stress to cope with and the child could withdraw from social relationships. This consequently may increase the strain on domestic relationships and the child may withdraw more, spending much of their time on their own. Whilst this example is an extreme one, it demonstrates the impact poor mental health can have on a child.

A positive and nurturing environment is key in reducing the likelihood of mental health difficulties for children. If children have experienced a poor environment in the past, this could be at home, perhaps if the child has witnessed domestic violence, or at school, the child could have been bullied, these events would have impacted on the development of the child and on how the child manages everyday situations. Evidence has shown that with children who have been subject to any developmental trauma, their brains develop much slower and are generally much smaller than children that have grown up in nurturing and warm environments (Perry, 2008). The differences in how children develop in relation to their positive and negative environments will be considerably different, thus high-lighting the importance to consider the stage of the child development rather than the child's chronological age.

Depending on the stage the child is at, will depend on their ability to manage group dynamics too. Participation can come in many forms, sometimes this is on an individual basis, sometimes this may be in groups. Managing groups can be challenging and needs specific skills and experi-ence to manage them effectively. When children are in a group together, ensuring that all children are able to have their say is important. Ensuring that some children are not dominating the group will take some careful management. It is important to think about how many children you have in a group and also manage the age ranges. Not having a too wide age range will be important for children to feel that it will be a permissive environment for them engage and not feel intimidated. It is suggested that having more than eight in a group at any one time will be difficult to manage effectively (Krueger & Casey, 2000). There are some fun ways to do this with children, so everyone has an equal opportunity to participate.

Fun ways to manage group participation with children:

- Give each child a number of tokens, each time they contribute they have to hand in a token. Once they run out of tokens they will have to listen to others. This helps everyone to contribute and ensures that the more dominant children listen to others once they have run out of tokens.
- Using the pencil technique, where the only person that can talk is the person who holds the pencil – this ensures that only one child speaks

at a time, the quieter children can still get to speak. The group facilitator can ensure that this happens.

- Use sticky notes for children to put their ideas on, this way everyone gets chance to contribute to the discussion.
- Split the group off to work in pairs and ask them to work together to provide answers or ideas. By reducing the number of people that children have to contend with will improve their participation.
- Ask children to work on, or suggest ideas for different aspects so that all children are able to contribute to the group.

The Impact of Neurodevelopmental Difficulties on Children's Participation

Neurodevelopmental difficulties are generally lifelong difficulties that develop from childhood. Whilst there are a spectrum of disorders, some of the most prevalent disorders that are known are autistic spectrum disorder (ASD), attention deficit hyperactivity disorder (ADHD) and tic disorders such as Tourette's (World Health Organization, 2010). Children with neurodevelopmental disorders are three to six times more likely to have a mental health disorder than the general population (King's College London, 2022). These disorders and their associated difficulties become more evident in different aspects of life. ASD is a disorder that is diagnosed through having specific challenges in three domains, these are social interaction, social communication, and imagination (ASD helping hands, 2022). There are many children who may have difficulties in one or two of the domains of the ASD triad, but these children would not meet the criteria for having ASD but would be considered as having ASD traits. Children with ASD generally find it difficult to make and maintain friendships, they can find it difficult to interact socially. Autistic children also think quite logically and so abstract concepts can be difficult to understand. However, there are positive aspects for children with ASD, as they can be gifted in talents, such as being able to sing, play musical instruments or draw extremely well. Autistic children can also have a good mind for numbers and dates and so can be excellent mathematicians and historians.

When involving children with ASD in participation, building on the child's strengths and understanding the child's needs beforehand will be helpful. How can you best involve the child knowing what strengths they have, for example, if they are good with numbers is there a particular aspect of the group session that includes numbers or maths that the child could be responsible for? Is there something that the child is particularly interested in that could focus the child's participation in the group? The child may find social interaction challenging and scary, so finding a way that you can involve the child without them feeling it is too challenging for them is imperative. For some children giving them eight seconds to respond to a question can be helpful. This is because it can take some time for children with ASD to process the question and to provide a response. Another way to support children with ASD in participation is providing the child with the details about what is going to happen in the group beforehand, so the child knows what to expect, this will help reduce some of the anxiety the child may feel; the phrase 'forewarned is fore-armed' is helpful to remember in this instance. Engaging the child in smaller groups could be helpful or allowing them to spend some time away from the larger group might help reduce some of the child's anxiety.

ADHD is an umbrella disorder that determines children to have difficulties with impulse control, concentration, hyperactivity, and organisation skills. Boys and girls can present very differently with ADHD, with girls appearing more aloof and having a propensity for daydreaming, finding it difficult to make decisions and completing tasks (World Health Organization, 2010). At times children with ADHD can struggle with managing big emotions and can lash out or become very distressed in a short space of time. It is important to know what strategies each child uses to manage these situations so a support plan can be provided for them whilst they are engaging with participation. Positively for children with ADHD, they can be very creative and 'out of the box' thinkers. They can have lots of positive energy and motivation to do things. Children with ADHD can also be quick thinkers and work well in pressured situations. Supporting children with ADHD to engage in participation requires the facilitator to provide clear boundaries and expectations for the child; including a space for time out may be helpful so that the child can manage their feelings in a less stimulated environment; providing this time out space may improve overall engagement in the group from the child.

Tic disorders come in many shapes and forms. One such disorder is Tourette's, where a child may be compelled to make repetitive movements, these can be motor tics, where the child may be compelled to stretch or twitch the torso, neck, or any other part of the body or it could be a verbal tic, where children are compelled to make repetitive noises, squeals, sounds or at times words. Tourettes is anecdotally considered by the public to be a disorder where children repetitively swear or hit out. Whilst this can happen with Tourettes, it is more likely children will have motor and verbal tics that do not include hitting or swearing. Children with Tourette's can have photographic memories and have good reflexes. Again, using the strengths of children in the participation groups will be really important to support the best engagement possible. In terms of managing the tics in the participation group, speak with the child beforehand and ask them how they want to be supported. Also ask about how they would like the other children to respond to the child's tics. Tics can be quite severe and can interrupt the child in being able to converse or think. It will be important that time is given for the child to communicate in the group, similar to those children with ASD.

In summary, for children with neurodevelopmental disorders the following interventions can be helpful to improve engagement:

- Give children the details about how the group is going to be run, what is the group going to include, how many children will be involved, the questions that might be asked, the tasks that the group might participate in, how long the group will go on for, days before the group commences.
- Providing a visual timetable for the group will help manage expectations throughout.
- Ask children before they go into the group the best way they can manage their condition and what help is required from the rest of the group. Find out what needs to be in place for the child to fully engage.
- Set the expectations in the group about how children should respond to each other's difficulties, this may benefit from a group discussion from the outset, setting ground rules and respecting differences.
- Give children clear boundaries and expectation for the group about behaviours and supporting everyone to be involved.
- Provide a time out space for children, so they can go to this space if they feel overwhelmed in any way.
- Allow children up to eight seconds to respond to a question in case there are any processing difficulties.
- Use children's strengths in the group to enhance engagement in participation.
- Use smaller groups or pairs in the participation group to help reduce the anxiety in the social interaction.

Communication with Children to Enhance Participation

We have already touched on some of the communication methods that can be used to enhance engagement for children. Using visual aids can complement the verbal message being conveyed. Think carefully about the language being used. It is very easy to use language that you think children will understand, however children can go through entire conversations without understanding what was being said (Cox, 2021). Using synonyms to help children understand the meaning of words can help arrive at an agreed definition if you are discussing something specific. An example may be, if you are talking about the word consent, then you may want to share other synonyms to help the child understand the context of the word, some examples are: allow; permission; agreement; authorise; approve; and accept (Lexico, 2022).

Visual guides can be very helpful in improving engagement in participation, we have discussed using visual ways of communicating previously in this chapter, using diagrams, pictures, and timetables to help children orientate themselves to what might be happening next. Or using more visual techniques to help children understand the overarching rationale for participation, for example, when services are asking for children to be involved in participation, think about how you are ensuring you are reaching out to children of all ages through the visual communication method that is being used. Using videos or animation will help children understand what is required of them or if children have been involved in participation before, they can share their own experiences to help other children understand. Having leaflets that children can pick up and read and reread when necessary is helpful to children in them being able to retain the information that is being given to them (Alderson & Montgomery, 1996). Giving information to children in more than one form is considered best practice, so that children can consider the information in different ways and over a period of time (Alderson, 2007; Bowers & Dubicka, 2009).

Personalisation is where the group is adapted to include the individual needs and preferences of children to optimise their involvement. Children need connection with others to fully engage with them. Building the therapeutic relationship with children is paramount for positive engagement in participation. Knowing what each individual child prefers, in terms of the way they receive information, the way they want to report information back will be important for the facilitator to know and include these methods in the participation groups. When children have a sense of connection, their engagement will improve (Cox, 2021).

Reasonable adjustments were an outcome of the Equality Act (2010). The Act places obligation on the employer to ensure that any employee would be provided with reasonable adjustments to undertake their work in an attempt to reduce the inequality for those with disabilities. Further to this it placed obligation on any services to make reasonable adjustments for their service users to access services. This would be the same for children who have a disability that require reasonable adjustments to access participation groups. Below are some examples of reasonable adjustments:

- Providing a seat in the room close enough to all members of the group where the child could hear properly.
- Providing the information on specific coloured paper to help a child with dyslexia to be able read it.

- Allowing a child to come in the room before others to help reduce the level of anxiety.
- Providing a child with a wheelchair-accessible room.
- Providing information in more than one format so they can process the information over time.

Providing reasonable adjustments is a requirement of law, so it is important that this is considered when facilitating participation, whether this is on an individual or in a group base setting. To find out more information about reasonable adjustments, review the resources here: http s://www.gov.uk/government/publications/reasonable-adjustments-a-legal-d uty/reasonable-adjustments-a-legal-duty (H.M. Government, 2022).

Overcoming Barriers for Children Maintaining their Involvement in Participation

There are always barriers to overcome when involving children in participation. Access is usually the first barrier; how do you get the right time and place to suit all children? Do children require a hybrid of online accessibility and face-to-face for example? Understanding children's preferences and providing different ways for children to engage will be helpful. The accessibility of the group for younger children is an important consideration. Reviewing style and content, such as using questionnaires, activities, and a more hands-on approach will need to be considered.

There is a need to think about the topics that are being discussed. Are these likely to be triggering for children related to previous distress they have experienced? Children could find talking about certain subjects too painful so it will be important to have an agreement in how, if this situation occurs, it is going to be managed. How will children let the facilitator know when they are struggling with a particular topic and how is that going to managed in the group? Are children going to be provided support at the time, or provided with a separate space that they can access, or how do they voice that they do not want to participate in that aspect of the discussion. It is important to understand the symptoms of trauma so these can be identified in the group by the facilitator and support the child where required. Having a trauma-informed approach to the participation group will be helpful, so that there is understanding and management of children experiencing trauma.

Parents and carers (hereafter 'parents') are an important part of children's lives and therefore managing parental expectations will enable the parent to support their children to engage better in participation. It is important to include parents, this does not necessarily mean that parents have to consent for their children to participate, but by keeping parents informed there is less likelihood for conflict and disagreements. If there are disagreements between children being involved in participation then there should be a policy or procedure that supports a mediated discussion between the child and the parent. If the child's involvement cannot be resolved at the mediated meeting, then other ways could be considered for the child to provide their views. This could be through 'you said, we did' boards, or through other feedback systems. It may be that the child could be given the information from the plan of the participation group and provide feedback on an individual basis, which may be more aligned to the parental views.

Consent for Participation

The legal frameworks around consent for children can be unclear at times. There are two main frameworks that you need to be aware of, these are Gillick Competency (Gillick v Norfolk and Wisbech Health Authority, 1985) and the Mental Capacity Act 2005.

Gillick competency is the framework that guides how and when children under the age of 16 years old can consent for themselves. Victoria Gillick took Norwich and Wisbech health authority to court after the department of social security disseminated a health circular about children under the age of 16 years being able to consent to having contraceptives without parents' knowledge. This would mean that parents would not have any jurisdiction to overturn the consent. This framework was initially established in healthcare law, but is now generally accepted across education and in social circumstances. The Gillick case was presided by Lord Scarman who stated:

> it is not enough that [they] should understand the nature of the advice which is being given. [They] must also have a sufficient maturity to understand what is involved.
>
> (Ibid)

The Gillick ruling does demand that a child understands the decision being made but also the consequences, benefits and risks in relation to the decision. Gillick does not specify what age a child has to be to make a decision, only that they have literal and lateral understanding of the decision being made. This means that children from a very young age can make decisions and consent to aspects of their lives if they can demonstrate competency to do so. There is also an importance to not burden a child with a decision that it is too big for them to make. For example, if it was a decision concerning significant risk, then based on the maturity aspect requirements of Gillick's competency criteria, you would not be burdening an eight-year-old with such a decision to consent to (Alderson

& Montgomery, 1996). However, what is important and a legally binding concept, is that all children should have their views and wishes heard and be involved in as much of the decision making that they can be or want to be, even if they are not consenting to a decision (Children Act, 1989; Human Rights Act, 1998). All children under the age of 16 years are presumed not to have competence or capacity, and therefore capacity has to be proved.

The Mental Capacity Act (2005) is a framework that guides capacity for decision making for anyone aged 16 years who are presumed to have capacity. Therefore, the absence of capacity has to be proved. Whether you have to prove that a child has capacity or prove that it is absent, the assessment is similar. This template below, adapted from Cox (2021, p.200), is a useful tool to use with children to ensure that the criteria has been met and capacity and competence has been proven.

If this template is used and each of the questions can be completed by the child, then this demonstrates that the capacity threshold has been met. Should any of the questions not be completed, then this gives the facilitator opportunity to improve the child's capacity and ability to consent by providing information and relevant detail for the specific question for the child to be able to answer the headings in each box. It is the responsibility of any adult working with children to improve the capacity of a child (Larcher & Hutchinson, 2009). By helping the child to develop

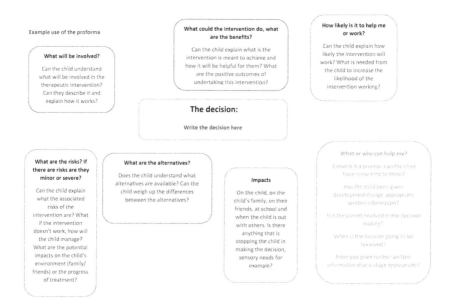

Figure 10.1 Helping a child form a view for decision making and consent
Source: Cox (2021).

experiences of making decisions, you are improving the child's heuristics for them to draw on in the future, thus supporting the child to be a better decision maker in adult life (Klaczynski, 2004).

When considering using children's consent for engaging in participation or for specific decisions whilst the child is participating, this should not be at the absence of the parent. Parents remain having rights for their child until they are 18 years of age (Children Act, 1989), however, once a child has got the competency and capacity to consent, parental rights become somewhat redundant. However, by keeping parents informed of what their child will be doing in participation, will support better collaboration between the parent, the child and the participation group. By not involving parents in the decision making, it is possible that parents will exercise more control and this may hinder the child's involvement in participation, thus making the absence of the parent counterproductive. Negotiation between the child and parent is critical to ensure good engagement of the child. The child can consent to take part, without parental consent, if they can demonstrate capacity. Once this has been determined, a discussion should take place with the child to ascertain how the parent can be informed and involved in understanding what the child is participating in.

Key points for children consenting to engage in participation:

- A child of any age could consent to a decision if they can prove their competence and capacity for the decision.
- The Gillick framework (1985) supports children aged under 16 years.
- Children under 16 years, start from a presumption of not having capacity or competence.
- The Mental Capacity Act (2005) is the legal framework for children aged 16 years and over.
- Children aged 16 years and over start from a presumption of having capacity.
- All children can be supported to improve their capacity.
- Parents should be involved or have an awareness of the child's decision making and be informed of what is happening with their child as much as possible. This must be agreed with the child beforehand.

Summary

This chapter has explored the impact of child development and the developmental stage of the child on engaging children in participation. The chapter has provided a range of strategies that support children with diverse needs, including poor mental health, children with neurodevelopmental difficulties and for those children who are considered having a disability and require reasonable adjustments. The chapter has included ways in which barriers can be overcome for the child and the parents. A framework has been offered to support children being integral to the decision-making process whilst engaging with participation. Finally, the context of children's rights in relation to consent has been explored alongside that of parental rights and how best to support a harmonious way forward.

References

Alderson, P. (2007) Competent children? Minors' consent to health care treatment and research. *Social Science and Medicine.* 65, pp:2272–2283.

Alderson, P. & Montgomery, J. (1996) *Health care choices: Making decisions with children.* Institute for Public Policy Research: London.

ASD helping hands (2022) The Triad of impairment. [Online]. Available at: https://www.asdhelpinghands.org.uk/supporting-you/information/autism/the-triad-of-impairment/. Accessed: 31 July 2022.

Bronfenbrenner, U. (1979) *The ecology of human development.* Harvard University Press: London.

Brooker, Liz & Woodhead, Martin eds. (2008) *Developing Positive Identities: Diversity and Young Children. Early Childhood in Focus.* Milton Keynes: Open University.

Bowers, M. & Dubicka, B. (2009) Legal dilemmas for clinicians involved in the care and treatment of children and young people with mental disorder. *Child: Care, Health and Development.* 36(4), pp:592–596.

Children Act (1989) London: HMSO.

Cox, A. M. (2021) *How can children aged 8–12 years be involved in decision-making and consent processes in outpatient Child and Adolescent Mental Health Services (CAMHS)? An embedded case study.* D.Prof. University of Derby.

Cox, S., Robinson-Pant, C., Dyer, C. & Schweisfurth, M. (2010) *Children as decision makers in education.* Continuum: London.

Davies, L. C., Williams, H., Yamashita. & Man-Hing, K. O. (2005) *Inspiring schools: Impact and outcome. Taking up the challenge of pupil participation.* Carnegie UK Trust: London.

Equality Act (2010) [Online] Available at: https://www.gov.uk/guidance/equality-act-2010-guidance. Accessed: 31 July 2022.

Erikson, E. (1980) *Identity and the life cycle.* W.W Norton & Company: London.

Gillick v Norfolk and Wisbech Health Authority (1985) 2 W.L.R. 413.

Hannam, D. (2001) A pilot study to evaluate the impact of the student participation aspects of the citizenship order on standards of education in secondary schools. Department of education and Employment: London.

H.M. Government (2022) Reasonable adjustments: A legal Duty. [Online] Available at: https://www.gov.uk/government/publications/reasonable-adjustments-a-legal-duty/reasonable-adjustments-a-legal-duty. Accessed: 31 July 2022.

Human Rights Act (1998) [Online]. Available at: http://www.legislation.gov.uk/ukpga/1998/42/crossheading/public-authorities. Accessed: 31 July 2022.

King's College London (2022) Mental health problems in neurodevelopmental disorders. [Online] Available at: https://www.kcl.ac.uk/research/mental-health-problems-in-neurodevelopmental-disorders. Accessed: 31 July 2022.

Klaczynski, P. A. (2004) A dual process of adolescent development. Implications for decision-making, reasoning and identity. In: Kail, R. V. (Ed.) *Advances in child development and behaviour.* 32, pp.73–123. Academic Press: Oxford.

Kreuger, R. A., & Casey, M. A. (2000) *Focus groups: A practical guide for applied research.* Sage: London.

Larcher, V. & Hutchinson, A. (2010) How should paediatricians assess Gillick competence? *Archives of Disease in Childhood.* 95, pp:307–311.

Lexico (2022) Consent. [Online] Available at: https://www.lexico.com/synonyms/consent. Accessed: 30 July 2022.

Lindahl, Kristinm, Malik, Neenam, Kaczynski, Karen, *et al.* (2004) Couple Power Dynamics, systemic family functioning, and child adjustment: A test of a mediational model in a multiethnic sample. *Development and Psychopathology.* 16(3).

Maslow, A. H. (1943) A theory of human motivation. *Psychological Review.* 50, pp.370–396.

Mental Capacity Act (2005) [Online]. Available at: http://www.legislation.gov.uk/ukpga/2005/9/section/4. Accessed: 31 July 2022.

Moss, S. (2012) *Natural childhood.* The National Trust. Park Lane Press: London.

Perry, B. D. (2008) Child maltreatment: A neurodevelopmental perspective on the role of trauma and neglect in psychopathology. [Online] Available at: https://www.childtrauma.org/_files/ugd/aa51c7_6b493f28b1b74a95aae35bcd4fe807a5.pdf. Accessed: 30 July 2022.

Peterson, A. L. (2022) Mental health at home. Mentalising. [Online] Available at: https://mentalhealthathome.org/2021/10/08/what-is-mentalization/#:~:text=Mentalizing%20is%20the%20ability%20to%20capture%20those%20in,imagination.%20There%20are%20both%20interpersonal%20and%20self-reflective%20components. Accessed: 30 July 2022.

Piaget, J. (1964) Part I: Cognitive development in children – Piaget development and learning. *Journal of Research in Science Teaching.* 0(nS1), pp. S8–S18.

Ruddock, J & McIntyre, D. (2007) *Improving learning through consulting with pupils.* Routledge: London.

Tan, J. O. A. & Fegert, J. M. (2004) Capacity and competence in child and adolescent psychiatry. *Health Care Analysis.* 12(4), pp.285–294.

World Health Organization (2010) International Classification of Diseases 10. [Online] Available at: https://icd.who.int/browse10/2010/en. Accessed: 31 July 2022.

Xun Kuang (230–312 BC) Tell me and I forget, teach me and I may remember, involve me and I learn. *Goodreads.* [Online]. Available at: https://www.goodreads.com/quotes/7565817-tell-me-and-i-forget-teach-me-and-i-may#:~:text=%E2%80%9CTell%20me%20and%20I%20forget%2C%20teach%20me%20and,from%20there.%20The%20quote%20comes%20from%20the%20Xunzi. Accessed: 25 September 2022.

Chapter 11

Engaging with Diverse Communities

Amari Creak (They/Them), Harry Dixon (He/Him) and Zaynab "ZeZe" Sohawon (She/Her)

Introduction

The NHS constitution places equality and diversity at its core. It commits to an NHS accessible to all, based on need not background. It puts the patient at the centre of their care, necessitating that their own unique needs are taken into account – this includes any protected characteristics they may have. Most powerfully, it states: "We maximise our resources for the benefit of the whole community, and make sure nobody is excluded, discriminated against or left behind" (NHS England, 2021). This commitment isn't unique to the United Kingdom. The World Health Organization constitution (1946) states that "the highest attainable standard of health [is] a fundamental right of every human being". Engaging with diverse communities is therefore a core consideration services must make.

This chapter presents the thoughts of three different authors on how services can better engage with diverse communities. Our contributions differ in style, some are more traditionally academic than others. But we wish to highlight that this doesn't mean some are of a higher quality than others. Our styles reflect our experiences in mental health services and what we are comfortable sharing. Some are perhaps more political than others too. The aim of this chapter is simply to give you food for thought relating to how you engage with diverse communities. As discussed in the next section, intersectionality makes it impossible for us to give you a guide of how you explicitly engage with each social group.

A Note on Intersectionality

In 1989, American civil rights activist and academic Kimberlé Crenshaw first coined the term 'intersectionality' in their discussion on black feminist theory (Crenshaw, 1989). Crenshaw argued that the experiences of black women cannot simply be understood by the amalgamation of the experiences of black people and women, but instead must be treated as their own social group which faces unique challenges. Therefore, in order

DOI: 10.4324/9781003288800-11

to understand the experience of black women, one must engage with black women themselves, not just draw conclusions from the experiences of the black community or female community. Crenshaw's theory has become the lens through which modern-day scholars hold discussions surrounding gender, race, class, and sexuality (Cooper, 2015). The experiences of a young, Asian, gay, cisgendered male will be different to that of a woman of the same character. In the same way, when any one of those characteristics changes – for example to a white, gay, cisgendered male – their experiences based on their identity change too.

We wish to raise this point here as a criticism of the chapter that follows. We have divided the discussion in this chapter to surround three main groups; the LGBTQ+ community, young men, and the BIPOC (Black, Indigenous and People of Colour) community. Our first criticism of our own work is this division itself. When we consider intersectionality, it is impossible to understand the experiences of any individual based solely on their status as a cisgendered man, for example. Our second criticism, is the grouping of the BIPOC population as one category. Our author identifies as being from the South Asian community, but her experiences as a South Asian female will differ dramatically from that of an African American female. The same argument could be applied to our grouping of the LGBTQ+ community. Thirdly, we haven't included every group we possibly could here – for example, we do not include a section on physical disability. The reason we have done this is threefold. Firstly, these are the groups by which many organisations classify their diversity statistics and are therefore the groups they are interested in increasing and improving their engagement with. Secondly, it would be impossible to cover the experiences of every individual in this book. Identity is unique, so experiences are unique. We also identify with some parts of ourselves more strongly than others. The aim of this chapter isn't to understand everyone, but to begin to explore how we can start to better engage with the groups we aim to improve our engagement with. And thirdly, we could write a whole book on this topic alone. We have chosen these groups as we feel they are the most under-researched and feel there are lots of good resources out there for individual's wanting to be more inclusive of other groups such as those with a physical disability. We wholeheartedly welcome further research in this area and for other authors to add their thoughts on how we can better engage with the groups we have not included in this chapter.

LGBTQ+ – Amari Creak (They/Them)

In defining 'LGBTQ' for this chapter, we follow the definition by The Center (2023):

LGBTQ is an abbreviation for lesbian, gay, bisexual, transgender and queer or questioning. These terms are used to describe a person's sexual orientation or gender identity.

The LGBTQ+ community is constantly evolving, growing, and expanding as the identities encompassed by the acronym become more normalised and less ostracised by society. New identities are formed every year, and pre-existing identities expand as more and more people feel safe and comfortable coming out to friends, family, and their wider support networks. In fact, in my lived experience, the percentage of people who feel able to state their true identity and/or sexual orientation is at an all-time high and this is an indicator of the huge progress we have made as a society in allowing queer individuals to exist as themselves. However, we are far from eradicating the struggles that those under the LGBTQ+ umbrella face on a day-to-day basis and, as such, it is hugely important to make an active and informed effort to ensure that these individuals have a voice within mental health services, and that participation groups do not isolate the community.

As a whole, there is a far higher prevalence of mental health difficulties within the community than within individuals who identify as cisgender and heterosexual (cis-het) (Town et al., 2021). In fact, one in three LGBTQ+ young people in the UK will experience a mental health difficulty, as opposed to one in eight young people in the general population who will experience a mental health difficulty (NHS Digital, 2018). This increased susceptibility to mental health conditions could be down to a number of factors – increased social isolation, invalidating experiences, traumatic experiences due to homophobia and/or transphobia etc. – but whatever the contributing factor, queer individuals deserve trauma-informed mental health care that understands that these causes may differ from their cis-het peers.

One of the leading explanatory frameworks of health risk in the LGBTQ+ community is the minority stress model (Meyer, 2003), which indicates that this increased likelihood to develop mental ill health is predominantly due to specific traumas that can only be experienced by members of the community such as internalised homophobia. This further reiterates the need for specialised trauma-informed care. However, this ideal standard of care isn't experienced by all those who access care. One in eight LGBT people have experienced some form of unequal treatment from healthcare staff because they're LGBT and almost one in four LGBT people have witnessed discriminatory or negative remarks against LGBT people by healthcare staff (Stonewall, 2018).

The only way to ensure that we reach a point where LGBTQ+ individuals feel safe accessing mental health support, and that the support is tailored to the unique needs of the community, is by involving the community in conversations surrounding essential changes within these services. Real, meaningful engagement with LGBTQ+ individuals, both those who have accessed mental health services, and those who were not able to when they needed to, is the sole way to determine flaws, improvements, and highlights of the systems and services that are currently in place. Similarly, within individual care, it is essential to maintain open, two-way communication when working with a queer individual as every person's experience regarding their sexual orientation, gender identity, self-discovery and coming out are so unique.

One of the largest challenges faced by services when recruiting members of the community for group or individual participation projects is breaking down systemic discrimination and power-imbalance that has historically existed within healthcare services. With almost a quarter of the community having experienced and/or witnessed a discriminatory event against their sexual orientation or gender identity within a healthcare setting, 27% of trans individuals having been outed by healthcare professionals, and the vast majority of LGBTQ+ individuals having heard of events such as these occurring, it is incredibly important to take historical discriminatory abuse into account when designing participation strategies. Acknowledging these facts then allows us to adapt services to create a safe space for participation to create real, meaningful change. For example, a participation group solely for the LGBTQ+ community, led by staff who are also members of the community or are, at the least, extremely LGBTQ+ competent, is far more likely to reassure members that they are in a space where they are safe to share their true opinions. Similarly, within individual participation, peer support has been shown to be extremely beneficial in allowing members of the community to express their real thoughts on the treatment because LGBTQ+ peer workers "naturally enable mutual aid, as processing similar experiences allows for external validation and helps challenge negative self-beliefs" (Levenson et al., 2021).

Another obstacle to effective inclusion of the queer community in participation is the avoidance of 'tick-box' participation. Often, services become afraid of 'doing the wrong thing' when involving LGBTQ+ voices and, as such, either avoid inclusion altogether or including members of the community because they feel they have to and not because they intend on using these members to implement meaningful change within the service. In order to combat this, it is essential that services are clear from the offset what it is that they actually intend to achieve. In doing this, it allows participation to be targeted, effective, and validating to those who partake.

This is not an exhaustive list of obstacles by any means, but the practice behind overcoming these challenges, and indeed behind ensuring safe and meaningful inclusion, is the same. Listen to LGBTQ+ voices and uplift them, set realistic goals and plan around the aims, ensure that there is an intersectional approach to diversity, and consider past experiences of both the community and the individual have had in order to make sure that their safety comes before anything else.

Young Men – Harry Dixon (He/Him)

As a young cis-gendered male, I have experienced some great participation opportunities within children's mental health services and I have seen some real changes being made being led by children and young people, I have also experienced being tokenised, feeling pressured to agree with pre-made decisions and to also represent young males as a whole demographic.

Whether it's been government events, steering groups, tender bids, or a simple participation group, I was often the only young male attending these events, which proposed the obvious question, why? Are there barriers that stop young men wanting to participate in these kinds of formats? Or is the lack of representation reflective of a low number of young males accessing mental health services?

> I think culturally young men have always struggled to access mental health services because of the lack of positive male role models who talk about emotional and mental health wellbeing. If a young man struggles to identify their emotions, when they struggle and how and where to go to this provides the first barriers to them even getting into a support service. Once in service young males are often allocated female workers whom make up the majority of mental health services and this can feel like a disconnect to them and their identity. Young men have been taught through generations that to ask for help is seen as sign of weakness and they should 'just get on with it'. I have met countless young men who when actually accessing support feel ashamed to admit their difficulties and this shame is a barrier in itself.
> Children and Young People's Mental Health (CYPMH) service lead

Addressing these preconceived ideas and theories around why there might be barriers for young males accessing mental health services is a good place to start when trying to find solutions, but is the true number of young males who do not feel that they can report emotional, or wellbeing difficulties being reflected accurately?

> Analysis by different socio-demographic groups suggests that female respondents were more likely to report concern about the impact of the pandemic on their mental health (62%) than were males (40%).
> (Department for Education, 2022)

From having my own lived experience of access to inpatient children's mental health services, it was predominantly females who were my peers as service users, the few other males that were also there all had one thing in common, their behaviour in the community had been the main cause of what had led them to being in the inpatient setting, some with police involvement. One particularly ended up with a diagnosis of Autistic Spectrum Disorder after leaving the inpatient ward (following a two-year stint) and had reflected that the delay was due to him not having "typical male traits" of ASD. I was often compared to my female counterparts and was told by professionals that I was not prioritised due to the females having other physical symptoms that were being monitored, such as menstrual cycles. I often wondered why the male patients were often seen as more problematic and struggling with behavioural issues as opposed to being given the same empathic and caring approach to treatment as the female patients, and if this was just my experience or if it highlighted a bigger issue.

In my experience, males are consistently more likely to be reported as having a possible mental disorder in the attentional and behavioural difficulties, and that this is a growing number, which is widening the gap between males and females.

Being someone who has been quite active in participation events and speaking engagements for mental health services, I have fallen into the pattern of repeating my own life story, both highlighting and critiquing different parts of children's mental health services and advising on areas of improvement. I have always felt very privileged to be attending these events and being given a platform to share my story, I was often the only young person or previous service user speaking at these events and it became the running joke that the "Q+A" panel would just be questions directed at myself and no other panel members, mainly because I was a young male with lived experience of accessing services.

Some of these "questions" were just emotional responses from my talk, which I appreciated but at the same time felt confused by, or I would be compared to someone in the attendee's life who they related to me, but often, I would be asked questions that felt quite weighted with responsibility that would be served as advice for how different services would change their future approach to service users, either males specifically, or young people as a whole. It was a lot of pressure to speak on behalf of a whole gender or generation, but I always tried to answer and remind attendees that my experience, was no one else's exact experience, and the true core of any mental health practitioners work should be person-centred care.

Mental health services are far too clinical and lack engaging with young people in general in environments that feel safe and comfortable to them. Some young men I have worked with are happier and engage better when we have gone for a game of pool, football or boxing. We need to meet young people where THEY are at and not expect them to meet us and sit across a table from us… within the male cohort services and professionals need to be aware and respect that there are sub-cultures. Not all males enjoy sports, not all males are 'alpha types'.

CYPMH service lead

The future of children's mental health services does seem more adaptable and hopeful than ever, with more Mental Health Support Teams (MHST) being implemented across educational settings throughout the country, trying to tackle the lack of early help and preventative services that have been a trend of the past, more youth working projects are being commissioned to give more young people opportunities to engage in social activities and provide potential work opportunities locally and without cost, but the battle is far from over, only future reports and research into how many young people, and specifically males are accessing mental health services or are falling through the gaps. Adaptability and person-centred care is key.

BIPOC – Zaynab "ZeZe" Sohawon (She/Her)

Cultural competency can never be fully achieved. What I mean by cultural competency is being fully able to appreciate and walk the path of a young person in mental health participation who is a person of colour.

If you are still calling us BAME (Black, Asian and Minority Ethnic), you are already failing to value lived experience of BIPOC young people. When I have voiced this in participation settings, I am met with awkward conversations and deflective speeches because it embarrasses clinicians and policy makers to recognise us as non-white.

From the term of BAME, to the way that systems are set up, the participation service in youth mental health I feel are failing BIPOC young people. I am a young person with lived experience of psychosis, autism and personality disorder. I was subject to trauma in the manner of an exorcism due to my South Asian family misunderstanding my self harm for me being possessed. I was not possessed, just unwell. Often when I speak about my experiences within participation, most clinicians and policy makers are shocked that this happened. They are shocked because of being sheltered by the Western system of mental health treatment. This kind of phenomena is not unique to just me. Many BIPOC young people I met in the psychiatric inpatient system were not recognised as being poorly by mental health services because of their cultural communities. In turn, they would show up with me in psychiatric intensive care units as being severely psychotic or extremely manic. Often, early intervention and prevention in mental health services is specific only to non-BIPOC communities.

The participation system is not built to honour the role of lived experience of a BIPOC young person. Many young people in participation who share their lived experience in senior political roles are not people who look like me. In turn, there is a perpetuating cycle of BIPOC young people not having their voice heard in senior participation boards. As a TEDx speaker and charity founder, I have worked my way to make a difference to youth mental health participation. I can safely say that I can count on one hand how many BIPOC youth mental health advocates there are. As for white counterparts, there are countless. After a few years in advocacy, I convinced myself it was because I was just particularly good at articulating myself. I ignored the niggling feeling of being isolated. I continually asked myself, why am I seeing so few BIPOC advocates? Why do I feel isolated? Why is there nobody here who looks like me? However I know this not to be true. It is really because BIPOC young people do not access the same opportunities. We do not access mental health services in a successful or timely manner. So it makes sense why we don't access advocacy opportunities because it is not known to us that its an option. Many BIPOC young people slip under the radar for mental health services, hidden by culture and rejected by statutory services. Mental illness naturally presents differently in our communities due to cultural needs. If young people are not accessing services, they are not receiving treatment. If they are not receiving treatment, they are not getting better. If they are not getting better, they are not knowing about how to get their voices heard in participation to impact change to services systems-wide. It is a vicious cycle.

It appears the system is flawed and there is no priority to be delivering care and compassion through a cultural lens. In youth participation I have found that what aids to mitigate this problem is to recruit participation leads who are BIPOC. They have a cultural awareness and are sensitive to understanding the strains of mental health services being unable to value BIPOC lived experience. Having BIPOC participation leads mean that it is naturally easier to have a basis for connection to potential BIPOC youth advocates. A basis of connection, meaning "I look like you. I am someone that gets it. I understand the battle for advocating for BIPOC youth mental illness. I will help share the load, lets connect". Having BIPOC senior leadership or policy makers involved in participation also helps with this issue of visibility in youth mental health services. Often having a BIPOC participation lead helps to build a sense of connection and provides a person that "gets it".

Lived experience working in participation is inherently different in BIPOC communities. In an international conference I was helping to organise, there was a scheme to allocate bursaries to young people who would not otherwise have funds to attend the conference due to circumstances of being in different parts of the world. The application process soon made us come to the realisation that a poorly written application did not equate to a bad application. Sometimes, language barriers can often occur in BIPOC young people, in a way that it presents as if the young person is poor in advocacy. This is not the case. To meet this need, interpreters should be provided and language barriers acknowledged. A poor grasp of language does not mean poor advocacy, it means a different way of communicating.

Most BIPOC youth do not engage in participation boards, such as within the NHS, because this is not our typical place to hang out. If you want to source BIPOC youth, it starts within cultural communities, mosques, churches, temples. This is how services can achieve inclusivity and cultural understanding.

In participation, BIPOC is valued, but for all the wrong reasons. We are valued by systems because it appears the service is diverse and reaching out to marginalised demographics. It is a tokenistic exercise. Why BIPOC youth should really be valued is because we accessed services in a delayed fashion when we were at breaking point. We usually have experience of racism, adding another layer of complex trauma. We provide a unique experience due to being undervalued, but oversold. I have been to meetings where I have felt isolated and uncomfortable due to being the only brown person there. I was put on a pedestal and told it was brilliant that I brought a different perspective. There is an unspoken but natural assumption that we have to speak of racial trauma and cultural imbalances within mental health services if we are BIPOC. To encourage good practice, it is important to seek out specifically BIPOC individuals and communicate genuine interest in their experiences, whether it is of a racial experience or not. Value a BIPOC young person for all of their experiences, regardless of class.

Maltreatment based upon societal class does not extend to only BIPOC young people. It includes all layers of intersectionality, young people who are care-experienced care leavers, those who have suffered homelessness and those of a less financially able background. The struggles that these particular young people face are barriers to engagement and meaningful participation. Class plays a part in BIPOC young people. The "cure" for this is to actively seek these communities. It is common to find advertisements for participation for those who are BIPOC, but less common with young people from a less affluent background, who, for example, have grown up on a rough council estate. These young people deserve to be heard and for their advocacy to be championed.

Conclusion

We hope this chapter has given you some areas to think about when it comes to engaging with diverse communities. Our most important message is – we are not all the same. But there are things you can do to make participation more inclusive for all. Consider who you are not engaging with and why that might be the case. Consider our backgrounds and how that impacts on our stories. Lead with principle of trauma-informed care. Finally, know that while our stories and messages are unique, they include aspects experienced by other young people too. We don't speak for everybody, but we are not alone in our experiences.

References

Cooper, Brittney (2015) "Intersectionality", in Lisa Disch, and Mary Hawkesworth (eds), *The Oxford Handbook of Feminist Theory*, Oxford Handbooks (2016; online edn, Oxford Academic, 6 Jan. 2015). Available at: https://doi.org/10.1093/oxfordhb/9780199328581.013.20.

Crenshaw, K. (1989) "Demarginalizing the Intersection of Race and Sex: A Black Feminist Critique of Antidiscrimination Doctrine, Feminist Theory and Antiracist Politics", *University of Chicago Legal Forum*, 1989(1), pp. 139–167.

Department for Education (2022) State of the nation 2021: children and young people's wellbeing Research report. [online] Government Social Research, pp.65, 66, 76. Available at: https://assets.publishing.service.gov.uk/government/uploads/system/uploads/attachment_data/file/1053302/State_of_the_Nation_CYP_Wellbeing_2022.pdf [Accessed 20 July 2022].

Levenson, J. S., Craig, S. L. and Austin, A. (2021) "Trauma-informed and affirmative mental health practices with LGBTQ+ clients", *Psychological Services* [Preprint]. Available at: https://doi.org/10.1037/ser0000540.

Meyer, I. H. (2003) "Prejudice, social stress, and Mental Health in lesbian, gay, and bisexual populations: Conceptual issues and research evidence", *Psychological Bulletin*, 129 (5), pp. 674–697. Available at: https://doi.org/10.1037/0033-2909.129.5.674.

NHS Digital (2018) *Mental Health of Children and Young People in England, 2017: behaviours, lifestyles and identities*. NHS Digital.

NHS England (2012) NHS constitution for England. NHS England. Available at: https://www.gov.uk/government/publications/the-nhs-constitution-for-england (Accessed: 26 October 2022).

Stonewall (2018) *LGBT in Britain*. rep.

The Center (2023) Defining LGBTQIA+, The Lesbian, Gay, Bisexual & Transgender Community Center. Available at: https://gaycenter.org/about/lgbtq/ (Accessed: 24 November 2022).

Town, R. *et al.* (2021) "A qualitative investigation of LGBTQ+ young people's experiences and perceptions of self-managing their mental health", *European Child & Adolescent Psychiatry*, 31 (9), pp. 1441–1454. Available at: https://doi.org/10.1007/s00787-021-01783-w.

World Health Organization (WHO) (1946). *Constitution of the World Health Organization*. Basic Documents. Geneva: World Health Organization.

Chapter 12

Participation in the Community versus Inpatient Settings

Hannah Sharp (She/Her), Trafford Youth Cabinet,
Carol-Anne Murphy (She/Her),
Lucy North (She/Her), Sarah Hutchins (She/Her)
and Leanne Walker (She/They)

Introduction

Learning from past examples and what has come before is a great means to develop and one way to do this is learning through case study examples. Case studies do not need to be perfect examples of how to do something, rather they present examples and offer a chance to learn, reflect and grow and can act as a base to build on or develop from for the future (Barnes et al. 2007: 183). Exploring people's lived experiences allows problems to be identified, solutions to be explored and ways to overcome problems to emerge. Below are five case studies written from both community and inpatient settings, bringing various perspectives, including staff, service user, and parent/carer perspectives, presenting examples of participation within the field. Following these case studies there will be a discussion of what we can learn from their content. This chapter therefore has three purposes, to showcase real examples of participation to allow the reader to learn from them, to learn wider lessons to take away relating to participation, and to hopefully spark ideas around future participation activities. In this chapter, both the term 'participation' and 'co-production' are used to reference different levels of collaborative working.

Case Study 1: Community Participation with Service Users and Non-service Users

Trafford Youth Cabinet

Trafford Youth Cabinet have recently been involved in a regional campaign to improve mental health provision in schools by writing letters to headteachers to encourage them to think about how they can improve support for students. The idea came from discussions amongst a regional youth forum surrounding mental health and how young people can be better supported. Mental health campaigning has been a 'hot topic'

DOI: 10.4324/9781003288800-12

amongst our regional youth forum for years now, and multiple different campaigns have come out of it. What is interesting about our regional forum is that local forums come together to discuss issues and share ideas, but often this results in the creation of local campaigns tailored to the needs of each group's area. We are supported by youth workers, but we get to choose the topics for meetings and decide what we want to be involved in. We took the issue of mental health to the regional level, and worked with other young people to develop the project. We then took it back to our local level and worked to make it our own. This is true co-production: where ideas and projects are created and driven by those participating.

Part of our letter focused on improving early intervention services in schools. Not all of us has accessed these services, but we all had opinions on them. These opinions were built from experiences we've observed of friends, but also about what we would hypothetically want from a service we could access should we need to.

The experience was empowering for us. It made us feel like we were making a difference to a big issue. Though we are aware it only tackles a small part of the problem. We continue to campaign on the topic of mental health in schools because that's what we want to focus on as a group, not because we are told to focus on it by someone else. What we hope you learn from this, is that young people are capable of working together to come up with unique solutions to complex problems, and to enact those solutions. We also hope you learn that young people are capable of passion about policy issues; we aren't all apathetic. We have a passion for making things better and this drives us to create positive change.

Case Study 2: Participation in an Inpatient Unit

Carol-Anne Murphy (She/Her)

Within in an inpatient unit, there is what appears to be a 'captive audience'. The reality, however, is often very different. There are children and young people (CYP) there to collaborate with but it is important to note that they are there because they are unwell and maybe not able to consider different options. They may feel that their opinion is not helpful due to their depression and feelings of hopelessness, or they may be overcome with anxiety and not able to even think about the question being asked. Some CYP rely on their parents or carers making decisions for them when they are well and have not yet experienced being asked their opinion. Conversely, there are other young people who have almost been professionals when it comes to having their voice heard – they may have been on the school council, been a member of a youth parliament, or even advocated for their parent or carer as a young carer. Whilst they may already have skills in collaboration, the whole agenda should not land on their shoulders.

On speaking to young people who have had experience of being involved in participation they recounted that the saying "You said we did" should have been changed to "You said we didn't". That is rather telling and maybe more about the requests being made than the process overall. Other young people reported that staff appeared to be paying "lip service" to the idea of participation by having a noticeboard with ideas on, however this was not reviewed to see if the ideas had come to fruition.

The young people went on to say that when the unit was expecting "important visitors" then there would be a push to have the noticeboard updated with photos and quotes, which would demonstrate the role of participation. The young people, though, were keen to answer any questions in relation to participation in an honest, transparent way, which may well have led to some discrepancies for such visitors to untangle.

From a staff member's point of view, whilst participation is thought of as a "nice idea" it is often the first thing to be cancelled when other competing demands emerge. It is not often in a job plan therefore it is an "add on" to someone's already busy day. Staff have said that there should be a dedicated participation worker within a ward environment. It could be argued that participation is everyone's business and as such should not be the responsibility of one person.

In monthly community participation meetings – in this instance ironically with only clinicians present – there is a clear willingness to ensure the participation agenda is being addressed, but there are no additional human resources to do so. Whilst there is a budget allocated to participation, there is no clear shopping list. There is a view that all young people will want to be part of the participation agenda, but maybe we need to have them at the monthly meetings with the clinicians to be meaningful as there may already be a view that there is no point as decisions have already been made (in the professional participation meetings).

In a ward environment it is crucial to keep the participation agenda realistic. There is no point asking young people how they want to spend allocated monies without telling them how much there is. Likewise, asking them what furniture they would like – whilst taking into account risk management – can often help young people feel empowered, valued and safe – exactly what they are looking for. This, in turn, promotes trust, which then, in theory, enhances their whole therapeutic journey. Although this can and has been dependent on the underlying relationship between the young people and the clinicians working with them (Laugharne and Priebe, 2006).

Whilst there may be a real willingness to make participation meaningful, some elements of participation might be out with the scope of control of the community team or the inpatient team. CYP might suggest a change or have a great idea, but they may be hindered by the umbrella of Health and Safety. Young people who suggested a trip to climb mountains, when asked for summer activities, were not allowed to do this because of possible safety issues however the same group were allowed to go to the Lake District (another suggestion they had) and enjoy water-based activities. This did lend itself to discussions about boundaries and that is important to listen to, and plan based on young people's views, whilst reminding young people that they are part of a system that cannot work in isolation.

Feedback from a young person who has been an inpatient on numerous occasions, as well as open to community children and young people's mental health services (CYPMHS) for years, would suggest that without the therapeutic relationship, true participation does not happen. There can be a perceived power imbalance that leaves young people feeling that their voice is the last to be heard and is never quite loud enough to be heard. Although, conversely loud voices can be mistaken as angry voices, which on an inpatient unit could have unplanned consequences, which will completely detract from participation.

In previous roles, clinicians who requested changes/expressed ideas for improvement were often advised to get young people on board as their views were taken more seriously than those of the clinician. To some clinicians this was not true participation, but merely "ticking a box" and certainly not meaningful in any way. However, if, ultimately, the change would benefit the young person then perhaps this way was acceptable. An example of this was the updating of a waiting room, including a games console. This idea was thought to be negative as it might mean that young people would not want to leave the waiting room and realistically how long would they spend there if they arrived on time for their appointments. There was a definite no to the request by clinicians. However, when some young people wrote they would like a games console (in the comments and suggestions box), this was agreed with the rationale that it might reduce anxiety before appointments for young people who might be anxious.

Covid has provided different opportunities for participation being managed in a creative way. No longer should young people feel they have to come to a clinic base to be involved in shaping services and facilitating change. Technology has allowed the most socially anxious of young people to have a voice – a barrier to change in the past. Covid has also allowed young people to present their ideas nationally and internationally, as is the case of one young person who has overcome their anxiety and their needs associated with their neurodiversity met. This particular young person has helped the participation agenda at a strategic level rather than an operational level. Technology has allowed us a space to be creative and to perhaps enlist CYP who otherwise would not be confident to participate.

In summary, whilst CYPMHS are under tremendous pressure to transform services, the voice of the young person should be listened to and heard as a means of facilitating the transformation. Not just listened to but heard and responded to in a meaningful way both at an operational and strategic level. This should be the voice of all CYP with no barriers to communication in participation.

Case Study 3: Young People's Participation in Improving Assessment Letters and Other Communication

Lucy North (She/Her), People Participation Lead Norfolk and Suffolk NHS Foundation Trust (NSFT)

When people begin their recovery journey with NSFT, this starts with an assessment process. The assessment process sees the young person sharing with a mental health specialist what difficulties they are currently dealing with and how they would like things to be different. They work collaboratively with their clinician to determine what the best support will be. A follow-up assessment letter is then sent to the young person.

However, many young people began sharing their concerns as to the quality of the letters sent to them after an assessment. The letter outlined the conversation had between the young person and their clinician, including their presenting problem, treatment plan, and a crisis and safety plan. They shared that the poor letters meant they felt less able to trust their mental health service. They were also put off seeking further support in their recovery journey, which had a fundamental effect on their mental health. Staff also added their own similar views, saying the letters were inconsistent, of varying quality, with different layouts and information included depending on who was sending them.

A quality improvement project began in May 2021 with the Great Yarmouth and Waveney Youth Mental Health Team, which is a part of NSFT. The aim of the project was by February 2022 to consistently meet the co-produced letter standards, as measured by a bi-weekly-sampled audit, and to see a 70% improvement in quality. The initial measures of the project, formulated using quality improvement methodology, were:

- Bi-monthly audit of progress against quality standards.
- Balance measure – if assessment numbers increase, is this reflected in the quality audit?
- Taking a snapshot of the average length of time taken for assessment letters to be sent after the assessment.
- Speaking to young people.

The project team consisted of a people participation lead, young people's participation group members, clinical team leader, occupational therapist, mental health nurse, mental health practitioner, assistant practitioner, clinical support team administrator, data technician, general practitioner, clinical psychologist, principal psychologist, and was supported by a quality improvement coach.

Young People's Participation

Young people aged 14–25 were involved in the quality improvement project via the Young People's Participation Group. This is a group for those with lived experiences of mental health recovery or with experience caring for someone going through their own recovery.

In alignment with the People Participation Strategy (NSFT, 2021) to ensure "participation will be inclusive, equitable and accessible to all", there were a number of different opportunities for young people to share their feedback throughout the project, including the participation group, one-to-one conversations with the people participation lead, email, and text message.

At the start of the project, young people were initially consulted on their experiences of receiving assessment letters and shared their feedback:

> It feels at times the information could be inaccurate and stuff hadn't been said which felt like it was fitting the clinician's narrative. It didn't accurately capture the conversation.

There were a number of young people who could not recall receiving copies of their assessment letter. Those who had received copies shared that reading them could be triggering, which means they brought on or worsened mental health symptoms.

> I would like to see a clear plan, paraphrase what was said with the plan or offer suggestions of what support is available to me.
> The tone they're written in and the language used can be quite patronising and not compassionate. It feels like it's forgotten that a young person could read it, and it should be written to them personally not the GP.

Reflecting on their own experiences, Young Person S shared,

> Due to the wording of the letters, it feels like you're not being listened to, like I'm lying about my mental health struggles, and I feel put down. When you read the letters back, they can put you in a low

mood. Sometimes the words that are used, or sometimes they have errors in. It feels very cold, and I feel spoken down to … The way that they are worded should make me feel like I can trust the mental health worker. The communication was just terrible with these letters.

Young Person S added:

They could be improved just by changing the language used and how it is communicated. Phrase it in a way that you actually believe what the young person is telling you. Acknowledge that you believe them and accept it. Take the time to make sure there are no errors. Big errors can make a big difference. For example, I received a letter with incorrect dosage of medication. I thought I had done something wrong, and I felt like a burden for troubling the GP and my pharmacist for having to correct this mistake. Include useful numbers to call, and what to do in an emergency and in an out of hours situation.

The key themes of the young people's feedback were then mapped into four areas (Figure 12.1 below):

1   What information is helpful to have in an assessment letter.
2   What information is unhelpful to have in an assessment letter.
3   How the letter could be formatted.
4   Language and tone.

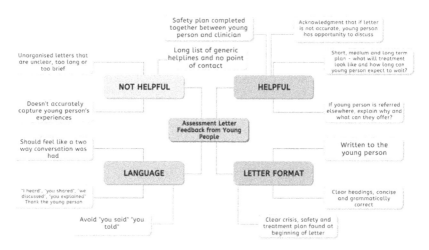

Figure 12.1 Theme map of assessment letter feedback from young people
Source: Author.

The initial themes from young people were shared within the Children, Families, and Young People's Community Mental Health Clinical Effectiveness Group. An update was shared through staff communication channels. The result of which led to some initial changes and improvements, including a change in language used and the formatting of letters, and saw the introduction of a working group for both parents and carers, and young people, to improve the quality of standardised letters shared.

Developing the Audit Tool

Staff worked alongside a local GP and young people, who were invited to review existing assessment letters before feeding back their views as to what was good, and areas where the quality and consistency of the letters could be improved. Eight young people reviewed six anonymised example assessment letters, provided through information governance to ensure they were appropriate to be shared. The letters varied in layout and structure, and demonstrated the current inconsistencies.

Examples of What Was Good Included

I like that the plans are at the start of the letter and are clear.

The letter is written to the young person and the language feels hopeful such as, "you've done well to keep safe" feels like they are saying back "we are going to help you."

They have given an opportunity to change the letter if something has not been recorded accurately and they thanked the young person.

The language and tone feels good. Phrases such as "you shared", "I heard", "you explained", "we spoke about," felt like the letter had been written together and not been done for the young person.

Examples of What Could be Improved Included

Providing a list of random [helpline] numbers to call is not helpful, I'm more likely to call someone in the service … or a helpline for something relevant to what I am going through.

Although I might live with someone at home or have friends in school, can I actually reach out to them for support. Don't assume because I get on well with my parents that means I can talk to them. A conversation should be had about support.

Should be clear and organised.

I'm worried that different clinicians are asking different questions so the formatting of the letters would be different. Standardised questions are good.

Following this feedback, the project team used the Plan, Do, Study, Act (PDSA) cycle as a model for improvement in co-producing an audit tool, enabling the testing of changes at a small scale (NHS England, 2022a). Young people worked alongside the quality improvement group to co-produce an initial audit tool consisting of a number of questions to determine the quality of the letters. However, during auditing both staff and young people felt the tool was not of a high enough standard to fully determine the quality of the letters. Through collaboration with young people and staff, the audit tool was revised (Figure 12.3) to be clearer and concise, with suitable headings and a change in the language used. It was important as part of the co-production process to take time to acknowledge that the initial audit tool was not working in the way it had been anticipated. It ensured the project group was able to pause and reflect together to improve the tool, even though this had resulted in a delay in progress. Using this tool, a baseline audit began with five letters using the scaling guidance as shown in (Figure 12.2 below).

The audit identified some key areas where the standards met were not at the expected level for young people:

- Of the eight letters audited, only half were written directly to the young person, and 50% had understandable and appropriate headings.
- Whilst 75% of the letters had a treatment plan, only two letters were rated *Gold Standard Plus* for clarity in what needs to happen now and in the longer term, with four letters rated *Totally Inadequate* and two for *No Entry*. Of those with a treatment plan, only one letter rated *Gold Standard Plus* whilst two were rated *No Entry* and one *Totally Inadequate*. Only 25% were found at the beginning of the letter.
- Some 25% had a safety plan and 25% had a crisis plan included. Of those with a crisis plan, 50% had no individualised information about

NA	0	1	2	3	4	5
Not Applicable Criterion not applicable to this young person's letter	No Entry Nothing recorded, completely blank, when it is clear that information is required.	Totally Inadequate: The quality is totally inadequate.	Poor Quality: The quality is somewhat inadequate.	Minimum Standard: Information reaches the minimum acceptable standard.	Gold Standard: Reaches all minimum standards and provides some minor points of additional information.	Gold Standard Plus: Far exceeds the minimum standard and provides additional relevent information on most aspects. Nothing additional/relevant could be added to improve the assessment letter further.

Figure 12.2 Scaling guidance used as part of the audit
Source: Author.

1. Does the letter have understandable and appropriate headings?
2. Plans **2.1 Is there a crisis plan?**
2.1.1. Is there individualised information about the young person in the plan?
2.1.2. Is it found at the beginning of the letter?
2.2 Is there a safety plan?
2.2.1. Is there individualised information about the young person in the plan?
2.2.2. Is it found at the beginning of the letter?
2.3 Is there a treatment plan?
2.3.1. Is there individualised information about the young person in the plan?
2.3.2. Is it found at the beginning of the letter?
3. Is it clear what needs to happen now, and what is the longer term treatment plan?
4. Is the letter compassionately written (is the language friendly, on the side of the young person and shows that believe them?)
5. Is the young persons voice present in the letter? (use of language a young person would have used rather than just professional language/avoiding clinical jargon)
6. Is the letter written to the young person?
7. Is the summary of the assessment written using the 5 P Formulation? (presenting, predisposing, participating, protective, perpetuating)
8. If any safeguarding issues have been documented, have they been done so respectfully?
8.1. Is it clear what actions were taken with regards the safeguarding issues documented, and why or why not?
9. Is the letter formatted so that it looks neat and appropriate?

Figure 12.3 Revised audit tool
Source: Author.

the young person and only one letter had the crisis plan at the beginning. However, of those with a safety plan, they were scored *Gold Standard* and *Gold Standard Plus* for individualised information about the young person and there was evidence they had been written collaboratively with the young person. Like with the crisis plan, only one letter included the safety plan at the beginning of the letter.

- When reviewing the language of the letters, five were determined to have *No Entry* when compassionately written, and the voice of the young person received four for *No Entry* and two for *Totally Inadequate*.
- However, of the five letters audited using the revised audit tool, 60% of letters were written using the 5P formulation (presenting, predisposing, participation, protective, and perpetuating).

Only one of the letters audited had a safeguarding issue raised, and was rated as *Minimum Standard* for having been raised respectfully and *Totally Inadequate* for clarity as to what actions were taken with regards to the safeguarding issues documented.

Finally, two of the letters audited were rated as *Gold Standard* and *Gold Standard Plus* for neat and appropriate formatting with one letter rated as *Minimum Standard*. Three of the letters were rated as *No Entry* and two as *Totally Inadequate*.

Reflecting back on the experience, **Young Person S** shared:

> Initially, I remember thinking 'I feel bad for the person.' But it made you want to do the best that you could to improve the letters. Although the letters were anonymised, it still belonged to a human being ... It made me feel really good that we were going to make these changes and that changes were going to be made ... It's helped to change the dynamic between the service user and the provider in only a positive way. I think sometimes service providers can feel desensitised. If they take five minutes to make these changes, they may be better able to empathise and be reminded that this is a person's life. It felt good to talk about the changes and I felt empowered. I could relate to those young people.... There was such a stark difference between the letters. They should be standardised across all of the mental health services. Why should only one mental health organisation adopt it when they all can benefit from it... It felt like I was making a difference and it was nice to see it materialise and raise awareness.

Co-production of Training

Young people in the project team proposed training to support staff members to improve the quality and consistency of assessment letters.

The project has been extended beyond February 2022 to allow for co-production of the training material.

To start this work, a young person, supported by the people participation lead, shared their own story and lived experience of communication from their mental health service. It meant members of the project team were able to hear a first-hand account of a service user's experience and reflect together before beginning to design an outline of the training.

The team agreed that key elements of training were to include:

• the young people's voice, including an open dialogue between staff and young people with key themes from the young people's perspective
• the administrative perspective to ensure letters are received in a timely manner, processed correctly
• an understanding of the impact on the wider professional system, such as GPs and other referrers.

Following advice and guidance from the Training and Education Department, the importance of all levels of communication were highlighted as a training need, including, but not limited to, assessment letters. In response, the project team are currently co-producing training to include all forms of communication, including phone calls, standardised letters, developing care plans, and communication within appointments.

A video has been produced to capture the young person's voice and to ensure that they will always be represented throughout training. Young people were involved in the development of the storyboard, the visuals and style and sharing how best they could share their story and voice.

Alongside this, a workshop was developed for staff to share their own experiences and what would be beneficial to them as part of the training. The feedback from both staff and young people has meant a template letter structure has been developed to be delivered alongside the training.

There is now a staff peer support group for colleagues undertaking assessments with young people who are supported by senior staff to review and audit their own letters together, sharing feedback and learning to improve the quality of work.

A further audit took place in June 2022 on 17 letters to assess the progress of the quality improvement project following the staff workshop and group. The audit saw an 8.87% improvement in the average percentage of standards met, requiring a further improvement of 25.49% to meet the projects aim of a 70% improvement in the quality of assessment letters.

Further key findings included a 15% improvement in the number of letters with understandable and appropriate headings. The greatest improvement has seen 34% more letters including a crisis plan. Eighty-eight per cent of letters included a treatment plan, an improvement of 13%, and 59% of letters were written to the young person, an improvement of 9%.

In September 2022, a snapshot audit was conducted with five letters, which saw the average percentage of standards met of 73.11% with 100% of letters written to the young person.

Following the completion of the production and delivery of training, a final audit will take place to ensure the project is maintaining its aim of a 70% improvement in quality.

Young Person S shared:

> The training and the auditing after staff have been trained, I think that the biggest thing now will be training and making sure it's implemented correctly... It gives me some kind of hope that services can deliver, and I hope that there will be more training and educating of staff.

Conclusion

The final word is left to **Young Person S**, who said:

> My hopes for the outcome of this project will be to make a positive change and will make a positive difference for other young people ... I'm hoping that young people will get the new letters and for them reading these will not be as distressing. I hope it opens their eyes; you might be doing it one way for ages but that doesn't necessarily mean it's right.

Case Study 4: Participation in the Community Done Virtually

Sarah Hutchins (She/Her), CAMHS (Child and Adolescent Mental Health Services) Expert by Experience (EbE)

Participation in the Community Done Virtually

The participation group discussed in this case study began meeting in December 2021 and it is provided in a community setting. In previous circumstances it would be undertaken face-to-face. However, in response to the COVID-19 pandemic, this changed to a virtual setting. When reflecting on the past seven months of running this group virtually, there have been challenges and benefits as well as learning to be shared, which will be outlined below.

One of the main benefits of running a virtual group, has been the ability to utilise online tools for collaboration. These can be tailored to the topic being covered in a group to ensure it's appropriate and to allow for alternative ways for young people to express their views and have their voices heard. This has been particularly useful for new members of the participation group. As we know, it can be extremely daunting to engage in something new, especially within a group setting. Therefore, being able to communicate using the chat function or via interactive whiteboards has been extremely affective when gathering feedback. However, a challenge has been finding new, engaging ways to collaborate online. It can be repetitive to use the same tools each time, despite how useful they have been in previous meetings. In a face-to-face session, there can be more activities and resources available to allow for free-flowing conversations about the topic at hand.

Another consideration of holding a participation group in a virtual setting is whether this is accessible to all young people wanting to engage. So far, the feedback has been mixed, but mostly in favour of a virtual setting. It has been highlighted that there is a higher level of convenience to be able to join the group from home, without having to worry about travel arrangements. It could be argued that it is more accessible for young people, as it means that there are fewer restrictions on the geographical areas that the participation group can cover. Nevertheless, the online setting isn't suitable for everyone – some young people have reported they would only be interested in joining in a face-to-face setting. There is a social and emotional limit to the connections that can be made in a virtual setting. This is an extremely important aspect of offering participation opportunities in a group setting. The chance to meet like-minded people who may have been through similar situations can bolster the group dynamic and lead to increased collaboration. It allows friendships to be built naturally and support networks to develop. This has developed in a virtual setting, but arguably not as authentically compared to an in person setting, due to private 1:1 conversation not being possible between the young people attending. In a virtual meeting, its often the case you are speaking to no one or everyone.

Example of a Participation Project Done Virtually

The participation group has been working on co-producing a resource, which will be distributed to young people newly referred to our local CAMHS. This has been a brilliant opportunity to shape the delivery of the service, at what can be a very daunting time for young people first accessing the service. It allowed us to speak with young people who have accessed the service themselves and ask them what they would have liked to know at this time in their CAMHS journey.

When the group was approached to work on this project, it was initially to gather ideas on the wording of an existing booklet that had been created by a CAMHS clinical team. Ideally, it would have been best practice to have the young people's voices present right from the start, but due to there not being an established participation group at the time, it was not feasible. However, it was quickly identified that the way we approached this within the group could compensate for that. Also, in this participation project, it did work well to have a starting point, which had up-to-date clinical information ready for us to work from.

This project was carried out completely virtually, and the use of online collaborative activities were extremely useful. The group used the inter-active digital whiteboard Jamboard (Google, 2022) which is free to use and allows for different forms of contributions. We first started by using Jamboard to ask the group to anonymously post via virtual sticky notes what they would have like to have known when they were referred to CAMHS. We then looked at the best way for the resource to be presented and method of delivery (e.g., paper version, via text or via a website). Having the option for the group to provide anonymous input online was extremely valuable and allowed us to gather in-depth ideas from all members of the group. We found this particularly useful when new members joined the group over the course of the project. Following this, the feedback collected was collated with the information which was in the original resource. Then, the participation group reviewed the clinical language to ensure it was user friendly and age appropriate and changes were made in line with the young person's views.

Jamboard was also used to determine the colour pallet for the design. In this activity, the group were asked to circle their favourite colours and cross out their least. Then, we all selected our favourite colours and luckily, they all went well together! We brainstormed which images we would like to use, via a virtual drawing activity. Following this it was identified that a young person wanted to draw an image that has been used in the final product.

The resource has gone through various internal clinical groups to ensure it contains the clinical information required before being printed and distributed. We received fantastic feedback from these groups on how the booklet will help young people and their families.

This project will result in a physical resource being created and distributed. Acknowledgement has been given, within the booklet, to the young people who were involved for their hard work and useful insights. We also provided vouchers as a thank you for their time. Throughout the group's hard work on this project, skills have been gained which could be added to the young people's CV's and applications in the future. It will also have a real impact on young people who are coming into the service by providing them with a guide on what to expect, who they will speak with, what therapies they might be offered and practical information such as locations and contact number. It has been a great project to work on, and the virtual setting has definitely aided the amount of collaboration that has taken place.

Case Study 5: #GettingThrough, Parent/Carer Participation at a National Level

Leanne Walker (She/They) – Expert by Experience on Behalf of, and With Thanks to, the #GettingThrough Team

What is #GettingThrough?

#GettingThrough (NHS England 2022b) is a series of guides co-produced with a range of stakeholders, including parents and carers and young people with lived experience, practitioners, NHS England (NHSE), and a designer. The resources are aimed at parents and carers whose child or young person has been admitted into a mental health inpatient unit. This case study centres on the co-production of the first of those guides, '#GettingThrough the first few days'. It was designed for parents/carers to fill out together with a permanent staff member within the first few days of their child or young person being admitted to a unit. The guide contains questions and prompts with space for parents or carers and/or a staff member to write answers. It is a conversation starter, helping to build relationships between parent/carer and the unit. It covers questions including 'where will my child sleep', 'how can I contact my child?', and 'when will the unit contact me?'. These are questions that the team found to be really important to parents and carers and yet were seen as unimportant or routine to people working in the unit 'in the know', and so were often overlooked or not discussed. For example, to a staff member it's clear where each child sleeps, but to a parent or carer who has never been inside a unit before, this is new information and it is not obvious that each child might have their own bedroom.

Background

#GettingThrough came from real experiences. The key message here is on being prepared to change direction. Originally, NHSE had engaged with parents and carers whose child had experience of children and young people's mental health inpatient units around service specifications and service design, with a view to undertake a different piece of work. However, over and over again what was heard was the experiences of parents and carers of not feeling included and involved in their child's care and the distress this caused, wider engagement events were then set up to explore this further. These events changed direction several times based on feedback in the room and then a small number of parents met and started to develop a guide, originally inspired by the practicalities and pragmatic approaches of airline safety guides and Council recycling guides ('you can put x in your re-cycling bin but you can't put y', 'fit your own oxygen mask first'). The team continued to develop the 'top tips' guide in conjunction with NHSE and was subsequently supported by the Children and Young People's (CYPs) Clinical Reference Group, as well as consulting widely with families and practitioners. A key element was to remember back to those 'first few days' and not to write from the perspective of a parent who had been engaged with 'the system' over a number of weeks or months. Emotion-free language and concise information were key. During the development process (which took approximately three years) the guide was trialled in units, went through various versions, was tested, brought to various forums and groups and every single sentence, word, and full stop earned its place.

Key Ingredients to Successful Co-production

Everyone in the #GettingThrough team was in agreement about this being a strong example of quality co-production. Interestingly, at the start co-production was not the sole focus or aim of the work (often people are invited to spaces with the intention of co-production with ongoing scheduled meetings). The approach was much more organic and due to that, the timeframes much more fluid and responsive (for example, meeting when needed instead of scheduled). Time was spent figuring out what felt right and which direction to head in. As a team, we reflected on the organic nature of the co-production of the guide and discussed why we felt that way, largely concluding three key ingredients, which created the environment. These were time, relationships, and skills, which shall all now be detailed.

Time

The space created to explore experiences and work was organic and was not rushed or time pressured, allowing the space to evolve. It would have been simple to say those lived experience voices at the start did not fit with the original project and then to move on, ignoring them or even to press on in a different direction regardless. There was also time to allow for the coming together of a range of different people, leading different lives. This meant being mindful and aware of different diaries and schedules, and arranging meetings for different times and days to include as many people as possible. To date, it has taken three years to get to the finished outcome. To some, this may feel like a lot of time, but the team are in agreement that the process has been just as important as the outcome. Past experiences of lived experience involvement had been described as having been commissioned for the outcome instead of the process with people running with ideas that did not work, just to get them done. The time allowed for the coming together of people to all learn and support each other to arrive at a product that worked for different stakeholders. This was important to build relationships with each other as a group, which shall be outlined as the next key ingredient.

Relationships

Through time, we had the space to get to know each other, as a team we strongly agreed this was fundamental. Mostly it enabled us to form genuine, trusting relationships where we could be honest and speak freely. We see this as crucial to the project as this enabled us to say things such as, 'I don't think that would work' and 'why don't we do this instead'. It opened this polite directness, which allowed us to explore freely what would work best. It wasn't just about having lived experience; it was about people being able to work together as a team in a way where each person could speak freely. It was the time to build these relationships, which led to the establishment of trust, which in turn led to giving up and sharing of power between NHSE and the team. We all trusted each other in what we were doing. When discussing relationships, we also felt lucky over the breadth of personality types that were involved. It happened to be that we all came together and got on in this way that empowered each other, true honest relationships developed where we began to get involved and support each other in other areas of work and life. This organic nature of the relationships was one in which the work was never more important than the people. The team also brought a variety of different lenses and skills, which is the next key ingredient.

Skills

As people with lived experience, in the project we were recognised as people with broad skillsets and encouraged to bring the breadth of our skills, knowledge, and experience to the work. Rather than being seen as just someone with lived experience. Through this pulling together of skills we had a diversity in knowledge and expertise to pour into what we were creating. The team reflected on how empowering it felt to be able to bring more than their lived experience into the project. It goes without saying that the team held such passion, driven by real experiences, to improve experiences for future families accessing care.

What Was Learnt?

Being such a strong example of co-production, does not mean the project came without its challenges or that nothing was learnt. Upon reflection, as a team we discussed two areas for future learning, these were awareness of diversity and what we have termed 'non-negotiables' and also reflected overall on the process.

Awareness of Diversity

Diversity was discussed a lot, especially at the beginning of #Getting-Through the first few days and it was felt important to have awareness around diversity in co-production spaces. As the guide developed, it was clear we could not claim to represent everyone (being a team of mostly women), but for example, although there were no dads on the core team, many knew what it meant to be a dad, knew dads, and had chatted to dads, and time was spent thinking about their perspectives and bringing examples to represent their voices. Wider consultation events happened to ensure diversity was represented in what we were doing, to engage in different perspectives as wide as possible. Alongside this, the wider diversity of experiences that were in the room at the beginning of the work was drawn upon. Towards the end of #GettingThrough the first few days, as a team we recognised there may be voices we still haven't heard and view this as part of the learning process, the test is in the using of the guide and constant seeking of feedback and amending to fit.

Knowing the 'Non-negotiables'

This is a phrase the team used to say, 'knowing the things from the start that are a must, fixed or cannot change, which we wished we knew before starting'. For example, there were governance structures that had to be followed, such as accessibility guidance around published documents in the NHS. These were things that the team did not have exact knowledge on, until coming upon a problem. As a result, a few times during work on the guides, where a lot of time was put into doing something, it was later found that it had to be done in a specific way. One of these specifics was font size, which seems like a minor issue but caused problems for the project. The #GettingThrough the First Few Days guide was finalised, which included formatting with a designer in an exact way with an already as minimal a number of words as possible. Upon going through standard NHSE publishing processes, it became apparent that the size had to go one up. This threw off the whole formatting of the document and led to further meetings to rethink, cut down and reformat. If this had been known at the start, the issue could have been easily mitigated against. The reflection being, we understood there were rules we had to work to, it was the not knowing them which caused problems.

Reflection on the Process

Overall, there is something important about not having such a spotlight focus on 'doing co-production', that allowed it to actually happen, organically. As a team we found an importance in the process of listening to and acting on lived experiences, which can have a positive impact for others and within that, allowing time in 'chaos' to allow for the direction of the work to emerge before jumping to try and fix or get to the solution too soon. There needed to be constant reflection and growth as a group. There have also been spin offs, which have come out of the development of the relationships within #GettingThrough, with additional projects and work together, this showcases the ripple effect of working in such an organic way.

Summary

In conclusion, this case study showed that with time, relationships, and skills, a natural evolution in order to find the best solution occurred. It was not about running with what others thought was wanted or needed, but developing based on real experiences and learning along the way. It was also important to have constant reflection and be flexible. The lack of direct focus on co-production, enabled co-production to happen naturally and the process in itself, in order to get to the end product, was highly important.

What Can We Learn from these Case Studies?

The case studies illustrate there is no one uniform approach or way to do participation, it looks and feels different depending on a whole range of factors including setting, local demographics and need. It therefore goes without saying, the case studies do not cover or touch upon all the angles, approaches or ways of doing participation but simply offer real-life examples to learn from.

Case study 1 draws out that participation does not have to involve children and young people who are currently service users. Youth councils and youth groups can be a fantastic resource for engaging with children and young people about mental health services. There is also an argument to be had about participation with children and young people who have had no involvement in services at all, which is also applicable to parents and carers of children and young people who have had no service involvement. Often, they will have friends, family members or know of people who have, or if they haven't, would still be able to think about questions such as 'if I do need a service/if my child needs a service, what would I want it to be like'. There may be reasons that children and young people have not accessed services such as them not meeting cultural needs (something explored in Chapter 11).

You can gauge what people without experience of services for whatever reason, know about services already and identify gaps that would make services more accessible to wider population groups. As highlighted by a

Trafford Youth Cabinet member during the collection of case study 1, a lot of the participation at the micro-level is the 'fight to be treated'. Young people are forced to advocate for themselves in order to get care in the first place. The young people in the midst of this 'fight' may not have yet been picked-up by services and therefore are an important group to engage with in service development at the meso-level too. Inpatient services could also learn here, that community service users can contribute to similar projects in their service. For example, the design of information that they would like to receive should they be admitted.

Case study 2 draws out the idea of children and young people's inpatient units having a 'captive audience' and an assumption that all young people will want to be involved in participation. Yet, some young people simply do not want to be involved for a variety of reasons. It also alludes to participation for show or to 'tick a box', but can result in positive consequences of change. There is also something here about culture around participation and maybe even raises the question whether participation is yet to be embedded fully and wholly into the children and young people's mental health field.

Across both the community and inpatient case studies, the importance of a positive relationship between service user and staff to facilitate good participation is clear. As part of the research for case study 2, feedback from a young person who has been an inpatient on numerous occasions, as well as open to community services suggested that without the therapeutic relationship, true participation does not happen. In the absence of this collaborative relationship, there can be a perceived power imbalance, which leaves young people feeling that their voice is the last to be heard and is never quite loud enough to be heard. Although conversely, and perhaps uniquely to an inpatient unit, loud voices can be mistaken as angry voices which on an inpatient unit could have unplanned consequences which will completely detract from participation and upset the therapeutic milieu.

Case study 3 is an example of participation being integrated throughout a project from start to finish. It demonstrates that young people are capable of being involved in what sometimes can be seen as complex parts of quality improvement projects. While this is a community case study, a similar method for involving young people could certainly be applied to an inpatient context. Young people highlighted a problem, NSFT listened and decided to act, they engaged with young people to further understand what was wrong and what 'good' ought to look like, and they involved them in evaluating the assessment letters. Participation does not end at the stage where young people make a complaint, to create meaningful change requires continuous engagement to fully understand the issue and create the change. Where this may differ between community and inpatient settings is retaining a patient group to remain part of the project. If an inpatient unit chooses only to have a participation group of their current inpatients, then discharge and transfer would disrupt the opportunity to have young people see the whole project through. This is where services perhaps could evaluate who they engage with and how. This case study is also important in that it highlights that participation can be measured and data can be gathered to evidence its success.

Case study 4 highlights that participation can successfully happen in forms outside of a physical face-to-face group and the use of online interactive tools helped with this. But it also highlights the inequalities this can cause such as access to the internet or a safe space to engage. The challenge discussed above around patient discharge and transfer causing issues retaining a participation project team could be overcome by engaging with patients virtually. Particular groups who would benefit from virtual participation in inpatient contexts are those who received a placement a long way from home and would not be able to travel to the service for in-person groups, those who may find it difficult to return to a service they have left, or those being treated in another setting, which they are not able to leave safely to travel to their old service. This case study perhaps also suggests having a range of ways that participation can occur is important, to enable more people to engage in participation in ways that work for them.

Case study 5 demonstrates how sometimes focusing too much on co-production can stunt its progress. Allowing projects to evolve naturally makes it easier for the involvement of lived experience partners. Like case study 3, lived experience was fundamental from the beginning. There are some unique challenges to engaging with parent/carers we can identify from the study. For example, engaging with parent/carers faces challenges with timetabling to a greater extent than with engaging with children and young people, but it evidently can be overcome. Part of this comes from paying lived experience members of the team so they are able to take time away from their standard day. Finally, it shows us how being clear on parameters from the beginning helps to aid the co-production process. These are all lessons that can be applied to both a community and inpatient setting.

References

Barnes, M., Newman, J., Sullivan, H. (2007). *Power, Participation and Political Renewal*. Bristol: The Policy Press.

Google (2022) Google Jamboard [Online]. Available at: https://jamboard.google.com/ (Accessed 14 September 2022).

Laugharne, R. & Priebe, S. (2006) Trust, choice and power in mental health: A literature review. *Social Psychiatry and Psychiatric Epidemiology.* 41(11): 843–852.

NHS England (2022a) Plan, Do, Study, Act (PDSA) cycles and the model for improvement. Available at https://www.england.nhs.uk/wp-content/uploads/2022/01/qsir-pdsa-cycles-model-for-improvement.pdf (Accessed 13 May 2022).

NHS England (2022b). #GettingThrough the first few days. [Online]. NHS England. Last Updated: 10 February 2022. Available at: https://www.england.nhs.uk/publication/gettingthrough-the-first-few-days/ (Accessed 8 August 2022).

Norfolk and Suffolk NHS Foundation Trust (NSFT) (2021) People Participation Strategy 2021–2024. Available at: https://www.nsft.nhs.uk/download.cfm?doc=docm93jijm4n1325.pdf&ver=1776 (Accessed: 23 April 2022).

Chapter 13

Peer Support: An Alternative Approach to Using Lived Experience

Oli Hawley (He/Him)

Introduction

It all begins with connection. That moment when someone else can show you that they understand what it is like to be in your shoes (Mead et al. 2001; Mead 2014; Nationell Samverkan för Psykisk Hälsa, 2016). You recognise that this person has experienced the same or similar pain, and the sharing of this so honestly and openly allows you both to be 'really seen' by one another (Brown, 2010). Not only this, but you can see that this person has been able to overcome these difficulties that seem so immovable, and this evokes feelings of hope that you too can get through this (Nationell Samverkan för Psykisk Hälsa, 2016; Watson, 2017). The person with you in this space is not trying to fix you or to compete with you. They allow you space to experience your pain in the way you need, and they give you permission to just 'be' (Mead et al., 2001; Mead and Filson, 2017). You can trust this person (Davidson et al., 2013; Watson, 2017). You can acknowledge that you are equals in this relationship, coming from the same place of experience and understanding wherein you are both the 'helper' and the 'helped', the 'giver' and the 'taker' (Faulkner and Kalathil, 2012; Mead, 2014). Through this symbiosis, you can become more comfortable being in this vulnerable space and can start to recognise and celebrate strengths and skills that you never realised you had (Mead et al., 2001; Mead, 2014; Watson, 2017). You can work with this person to grow and to learn together so as to move towards a life that you want (Mead, 2014). This is peer support.

As described by a research participant:

> It's not even about me needing to tell people my diagnosis or where I've been or where I've come from, but just being human. Shared humanity and sitting alongside people in wherever they are in their life has always been one of the most powerful things I found in relationships with young people ... we will come from this like compassionate place and this place that just says, 'That sounds really [awful]', that, you know, 'What you're going through sucks right now. That's okay'.

DOI: 10.4324/9781003288800-13

Research Participant

For children and young people (CYP), finding connection where they feel truly understood as their authentic self can often be limited to other CYP.[1] This becomes problematic when CYP struggle with physical and/or mental health difficulties as the professional support is typically provided by an adult. Not only this, but there is a culture that discourages mental health clinicians from sharing personal experience (Perkins and Repper, 2022) – the very vulnerability and authenticity that is prerequisite for that moment of connection (Brown, 2010). Perhaps the role of a peer support worker, who is themselves a child/young person, offers an alternative possibility for support, which can circumvent this two-faceted disconnect posed by child to adult and non-clinical to clinical relationship dynamics. To make this argument, this chapter explores what intentional peer support looks like in the context of children and young people's (CYPs) mental health services (MHS). It will consider the benefits, challenges, and realities of CYPs peer support through the investigation of first-hand experience of CYP peer support workers and parent/carer peer support workers, critically analysed within the context of peer support in mental health services. It will compare and contrast this to participation, identifying areas of overlap and difference, and will propose a synergistic relationship that the two disciplines can share moving forwards, affording greater recognition to the capabilities of CYP functioning as professionals within the mental health system.

Before we discuss and unpack the topic of peer support any further, it is important to note why it has been included within a book concerning CYPs participation. Participation and peer support are often misunderstood and conflated topics, being reduced down to 'lived experience of mental health challenges'. Not only does this offer little information, but it fails to capture the meaning and purpose of such initiatives. To be involved in participation/peer support is not simply to have experienced difficulties with one's mental health, but it refers to principled and boundaried approaches to drawing upon this experience in order to realise meaningful change. However, while there are many similarities between participation and peer support, there are also key differences, most pertinently in the way lived experience is used (explored later in this chapter and in Chapter 2). This chapter has been included to help differentiate between the two, while positing a case for peer support as a complementary and valid discipline in its own right. When well-defined and properly comprehended, peer support not only offers an alternative approach to using lived experience, but one that is symbiotic with the culture of participation.

What Does a 'Peer Support Worker' Do?

Peer support work can take a huge variety of different forms and practices, dependent on working context and the needs of the individual, team, and organisation (see Repper, 2013a). As noted by one research participant:

> We have to be very kind of on our toes with kind of just adapting to the young people that are in the room.

Research Participant

Rather than trying to create a definitive list, it is perhaps more useful to explore the fundamental commonalities between one peer support worker and another. These shared characteristics can be divided into three forms of inherent characteristics: *natures of being, natures of understanding*, and *natures of doing*. These three areas are not separate, but are the interconnected processes that result in what we recognise to be a 'peer'.

Natures of Being

The role of a peer fundamentally revolves around the drawing upon and sharing of lived and life experience: this is what sets it uniquely apart from other mental health practitioner roles (Mead and MacNeil, 2017; Davidson et al., 2013; Repper, 2013a; Mead, 2014; Perkins and Repper, 2022). This is to say, part of what it means to be a peer is encapsulated in their very nature of being. A peer is an expert in their experiences, having lived with mental health challenges of their own, or for a parent/carer peer, having lived experience of supporting someone else with mental health challenges. Their experiences with mental health difficulties will have shaped, and will continue to shape, how a peer understands and interacts with themselves and the world around them. They have felt the emotions, lived the challenges, and navigated the world through the lens of this mental health challenge: they have 'been' there, and some peers will continue to 'be' there as they pursue their own recovery journey. Intentional peer support allows for individuals to draw upon this lived experience as a tool to facilitate recovery of others, as well as themselves (Mead et al., 2001; Mead and MacNeil, 2017; Repper, 2013a; Fortuna et al., 2022).

Natures of Understanding

In a mental health context of peer support, 'nature of understanding' refers to the governing worldview and ideology of peer support that guides and delineates a 'peer' approach from other practitioners. Mead (2014, p.12) stresses the importance of a peer critically analysing 'how we've come to know what we know', particularly with the aim of unpicking the influence of psychiatric and medical models that those who experience mental health challenges can so easily internalise (Mead et al., 2001; Mead and MacNeil, 2017). Peers can instead bring about a perspective that places individuals within their larger sociocultural and political contexts, so that those who experience mental health difficulties are given permission to create and control their own identity, rather than to be pathologised and disempowered (Mead et al., 2001). Guidance for how to develop and embody the peer worldview is given in the form of principles by which peers are expected to act. Influential examples of peer principles are those of:

- Mead et al. (2001, p.135): 'respect, shared responsibility, and mutual agreement of what is helpful'
- Mead and MacNeil, (2017, p.6):

    a   'The peer principle (finding affiliation with someone with similar life experience and having an equal relationship),
    b   The helper principle (the notion that being helpful to someone else is also self-healing)
    c   Empowerment (finding hope and believing that recovery is possible; taking personal responsibility for making it happen),
    d   Advocacy (self and system advocacy skills), choice and decision-making opportunities, skill development, positive risk taking, reciprocity, support, sense of community, self-help, and developing awareness (Campbell, 2004; Clay, 2004)'.

- Repper's (2013a, p.8) eight core principles: 'mutuality, reciprocity, a "non-directive' approach, being recovery-focused, strengths-based, inclusive, progressive and safe'.

While there is variation in terminology, and this is not a definitive list of every possible principle/system of principles that could be included, the commonality between these three theorisations of peer principles offers useful insight into the peer worldview.

These principles can provide a useful reference point for how a peer may interpret and respond to situations, not a prescriptive list of linear tasks to be completed or undertaken. For example, understanding that safety is not the same as being 'risk free' (Mead and MacNeil, 2017; Repper, 2013a) provides us with a framework within which to work, but not a solution for how to approach every situation concerning safety. It must also be noted that a principle, 'a basic idea or rule that explains or controls how something happens or works' (Cambridge English

Table 13.1 Peer principles in theory compared to application

Combined peer principles	What this means for a 'peer worldview'
'respect' – (Mead et al., 2001, p.135), 'The peer principle (finding affiliation with someone with similar life experience and having an equal relationship)' (Mead and MacNeil, 2017, p.6), 'mutuality' (Repper, 2013a, p.8).	A relationship should be non-hierarchical so that both parties' contributions are of equal validity and importance. Connections should be formed on, and are made more meaningful through having shared experiences.* *Only related to Mead and MacNeil's (2017) and Repper (2013a), principles.
'shared responsibility' – (Mead et al., 2001, p.135) 'Empowerment (finding hope and believing that recovery is possible; taking personal responsibility for making it happen)', and 'self-help, and developing awareness' (Mead and MacNeil, 2017, p.6), 'being recovery-focused' 'strengths-based', and 'progressive'– (Repper, 2013a, p.8).	Recovery is possible for everyone. It is important to believe in the innate strengths, abilities, and capabilities of an individual; to focus on what someone can do, rather than what they cannot do. Autonomy and agency are important in recovery. Support to discover self-management skills and tools will empower the achievement of this.
'mutual agreement of what is helpful'– (Mead et al., 2001, p.135), 'Advocacy (self and system advocacy skills), choice and decision-making opportunities, skill development … reciprocity, support' (Mead and MacNeil, 2017, p.6), 'reciprocity', 'being recovery-focused', and 'a "non-directive" approach' – (Repper, 2013a, p.8).	Everyone should be included as much as possible** in any and all decisions concerning them. Being able to play a meaningful part of decision-making around support, including the determination of what is 'right' for them, fosters greater feelings of motivation than being told what to do (Deci, 2012). **Mental capacity must be taken into consideration: advanced directives and being knowledgeable about the person they support's wishes can aid with this.
'mutual agreement of what is helpful'– (Mead et al., 2001, p.135), 'sense of community' (Mead and MacNeil, 2017, p.6), 'inclusive' – (Repper, 2013a, p.8).	Recovery must consider the individual as a holistic whole. The overmedicalisation of those who struggle with their mental health creates an identity that revolves around being a 'patient', and creates a barrier that prevents them from connecting and reintegrating with their communities (Mead et al., 2001). Communities offer resources and support that are more tailored and it offers a needed sense of inclusion.
'positive risk taking (Mead and MacNeil, 2017, p.6), 'safety' – (Repper, 2013a, p.8)	Safety must be negotiated and mutually understood: it does not equate to being 'risk free'.

Combined peer principles	What this means for a 'peer worldview'
'The helper principle (the notion that being helpful to someone else is also self-healing)' (Mead and MacNeil, 2017, p.6)	The act of giving is beneficial in recovery.*** ***This could also be seen as an extension of Repper's (2013a) 'reciprocity' in that a peer gives to the relationship and also gains in return.

Source: Author.

Dictionary, 2022) is different to a competency, which Fortuna et al., (2022, p.580) see as the 'ability to carry out a specific role or function'. Competencies have been used as, 'guidance for training, certification and job descriptions' (ibid), 'to provide a clear understanding of how MH PSWs [Mental Health Peer Support Workers] add value' (Health Education England, 2020), and 'to protect people working in MH PSW roles from being asked to work in inappropriate ways' (ibid). These competencies may provide benefit and clarity to the organisation within which a peer works, but to define a peer by these would be to favour the efficacy of the role to its own ontology. Principles can offer guidance on a peer outlook, no matter the task set.

Natures of Doing

The 'nature of doing' refers to the key duties and tasks that a peer will undertake and collaborate on within their role. This is heavily informed by the nature of being and nature of understanding, and has been explored last so as to allow for the consideration of this.

Key Duties

- **Sharing lived experience to build reciprocity:** Peers make themselves vulnerable and relatable through the sharing of relevant parts of their journey so as to establish a mutual and trusting relationship (Brown, 2010; Mead et al., 2001; Watson, 2017).
- **Sharing lived experience to evoke hope and support recovery:** Through sharing lived experience, peers can inspire hope that recovery is possible, and model a success story for those they support, as well as staff (Davidson et al., 2013; Deegan, 1988; Repper, 2013a; Watson, 2017). Peers can use their understanding of recovery to support others to master their own recovery and towards the achievement of meaningful goals (Deegan, 1988; Repper and Watson, 2012; Watson, 2017).
- **Exploring recovery beyond being a 'service user':** Peers can help individuals to challenge preconceived notions of patient identity to

understand themselves in a more holistic, progressive way that facilitates a life beyond being 'mentally ill' (Mead et al., 2001; Mead, 2014).

- **Lived-experience-informed emotional support:** Through sharing similar experiences, it is thought that peers are able to more authentically empathise with these emotional difficulties and distress and can draw upon their own experiences as a tool to support those who are struggling (Mead and MacNeil, 2017; Scott, 2011; Repper and Carter, 2011).
- **Lived-experience-informed practical support:** Peers can support with everyday practical tasks, and may have expertise through doing these tasks for themselves, e.g., managing benefits (Repper and Watson; 2012; Watson, 2017).

These are a handful of typical duties that a peer will approach within their role, but is by far from an exhaustive list of specifics. What I hope to illuminate through this exploration of a peer through these different lenses is that a peer identity is complex and nuanced, and stretches far beyond the limited perspective offered by seeing it only as a role. A peer support worker is the title of an employment/voluntary position, but this must be undertaken by someone who lives as a peer and who understands the value framework underpinning the duties.

How Does this Compare to Participation?

Participation and peer support can be seen to begin from the same place: an opportunity for CYP to draw upon their lived and life experiences,[2] rather than taught expertise, as a tool for the benefit of themselves and others (Davidson, et al., 2013; Hart 1992; Mead et al., 2001; Mead and MacNeil, 2017). However, where peer support focuses on using lived experience to support other individuals, participation utilises lived experience to inform service improvement and development projects at an organisational level. Where participation initiatives would see staff educated around how to support CYP best, peer support workers function as this recovery-focused wealth of knowledge when they sit within multidisciplinary teams. The final part of the participation process is that CYP should reap the benefits of experiencing more CYPs-focused services. Comparatively, in peer support, which begins by offering a person-centred form of support, the final stage of their influence is the cultural shift and transformation through the dissemination of their recovery-focused approach. As such, we could conceptualise peer support as a 'bottom up' approach (Figure 13.1) and participation as a 'top down' approach (Figure 13.2) to culturally transforming Children and Young People's Mental Health Services (CYPMHS).

These proposed processes may demonstrate the similarity in transformative power that is held by well-utilised lived experience, in a MHS

Results in organisational and cultural transformation

Peers can have an influence on policy and procedure

Brings about a more recovery-focused way of working in teams which fosters hope and challeges stigma

Lived experience used to provide support to individuals accessing services

Figure 13.1 Peer support
Source: Influenced by Repper's (2013a) briefing paper.

Lived experience used to inform large-scale service development and improvement

Staff influenced through organisational change, trickle down learning and lived-experience teaching delivered through parcipitation initiatives

CYPs accessing services receive more person-centered and CYP-focused support through lived-experience guided initiatives and better trained staff

Results in organisational and cultural transformation

Figure 13.2 Participation
Source: Influenced by Day's (2008) article.

context, but it would be spurious to assume that participation and peer support are simply different terms for the same concept.

A further distinction to make is that of peer support vs peer support worker, and participation vs participant.[3] As detailed in Figure 13.1, peer support is a form of individual support that can be accessed to support with those who are facing mental health challenges. Comparatively, participation (Figure 13.2) uses lived experience as a basis for evidence and critical perspectives on service improvement. A peer-support worker could therefore be described primarily as, 'one who "does" peer support', and a participant could be described primarily as, 'one who "does" participation'. However, there can be occurrences where peer support appears within participation and vice versa. Peer-support workers have lived experience, of mental health challenges and sometimes of service access. They could be asked to participate within co-production/participation initiatives to contrast against the taught experience of other professionals involved. Equally, participants might find they have a tendency to more strongly empathise and know how to help other members of their group when they are struggling with their mental health – an informal peer support. Nonetheless, this does not mean that peer support and participation are the same, but rather that it is possible for peer support to facilitate the space to participate, and participation can facilitate an environment for peer support. It is important to keep a clear distinction between the two emerging[4] disciplines for the sake of ensuring safe boundaries, adequate support, and to maximise the capabilities for achievement through clarity of role and goal.

Children and Young People Acting as Peers

With much of the existing research in peer support centring on adults, an investigation was conducted to gather first-hand experience from CYP working as a peer for other CYP. For the purposes of the study, a CYP peer was defined as an individual between the ages of 0 and 25 who is working, or who has worked, as an intentional peer support worker for other CYP, i.e., they have occupied the position of peer support worker within a formally recognised organisation. The study looked to answer the question, 'How can the experience of CYP peers inform our understanding of the role?', with the aim of defining the key ideas that underpin the CYP peer-support process. Rather than taking an approach to consider how far CYP peers could be seen to confirm existing ideas and understandings, a more general, open-ended approach was taken. The hopes were for this to offer the opportunity for CYP to describe and explore what the role was, what they thought about CYP-to-CYP support, and to share their biggest lessons from working in this field.

The research approach taken was rooted in the values and approaches of peer support. This is to say that participants were treated as experts in their own experiences. The focus groups gave the participants the chance to find mutuality within their experiences, and it was topics that resonated strongly with other members of the group that would lead to further discussion, and as a result, to the generating of a theme. Participants were able to speak freely through the safety of a peer space and elements of humour, and taking and offering support around the validity of contributions could be found in the space. As outlined by Braun and Clarke (2006; 2019), thematic analysis approaches to psychological research recognise the active role that the researcher plays and while I recognise that I will have shaped the research process, I did not reciprocate within the space to avoid biasing the data.

This design and use of language surrounding the research paradigm was implemented because peer support by its very nature argues for the reconceptualisation and recontextualisation of how we approach the construction of knowledge. Peer support challenges the very basis of mental health support in that it argues for a redistribution of power from the oppressor to the oppressed and for a shift in focus from patient to someone who plays an active role in their recovery (Mead et al., 2001). To take an epistemological approach, which has an aim to discover universally applicable truths, such as positivism (Park et al., 2020), would be to ignore the very person-centred nature of peer support. As such, the research design could be seen to more closely align with the paradigm of qualitative research in that it looks to understand the individual subjectivities of the research participants and, in doing so, can build a larger narrative around how we might begin to approach CYPs peer work (Braun and Clarke, 2013). This study will not attempt to define a universal narrative, as this would be to set off to achieve something that disagrees with its epistemic foundations, but it offers a story of CYPs peer experience that we can use to further our own understanding, and to look to how we might continue to ask relevant questions so as to broaden this further.

The data in this study was collected from two semi-structured focus groups conducted over Zoom, the virtual meeting platform. Six CYP peers were selected for the focus groups who were, or had been, employed in charity and public sector organisations within England. Data was collected through audio and video recordings, and through downloading all data collected in Zoom's chat feature. The final transcripts were created by editing the automated transcripts in accordance with the audio and video recordings, and then interpolating chat data into the transcript, at the chronologically appropriate times.

A thematic analysis approach that drew upon the six stages of theme generation proposed by Braun and Clarke (2006; 2019) was taken. After familiarising myself with the transcription, I went through and generated codes from the data. These codes provided key insight into the larger themes at play and offered multiple possible groupings which, in turn, would produce very different overall themes. At first, I took the scope that these themes could be used to reinforce existing research and codes were grouped in accordance with peer values, peer skills, and organisational support. However, as the analysis developed, it became apparent that the best-fit of the code groupings generated themes of a real fundamental understanding of the core of a CYP peer role and its cultural positioning as a mental health support role. These themes were then tagged with direct quotes from the transcripts to allow for mutual ownership of the knowledge. The themes discovered were as follows: 'Being human', 'Be there with them', 'A stepping stone', 'Pay your peers', and 'The question of safety'. These are all outlined and explored in greater detail below.

Study Findings

'Being Human' – CYP Peers Connect Through Genuineness, Authenticity, and Relatability

This theme was generated from the idea that a CYP peer acts in a way that is true to them: they bring their authentic, holistic self to interactions which, in turn, builds connection with other CYP. As one person said:

> I'm chronically uncool, but I'm very much myself, um, and I think that's what young people respond to most is they just really care about you being honest and authentic and who you are.

Research Participant

The theme shows CYP need authenticity and relatability in relationships, and how there were feelings of alienation and disconnect towards those who could not demonstrate this. This experience of distrust from CYP towards services and those who work for them stems from the lack of knowing what it is like to be a CYP. Shared lived experience – having 'been' where someone else had 'been' – permitted peers to circumvent this disconnect and instead facilitated a connection based on shared vulnerability (a similar relational finding to Brown, 2010). The sharing of lived experience also served as a marker of CYPs peer's authenticity of self-presentation and as a way to prove one's genuineness of care for CYP. By not putting up a front, and bringing their full, true self to interactions with CYP, peers are seen as 'being human' by those who are supported by them. It is fundamental to note that there is not one way to 'be human' that CYP would accept, and it was actively addressed as a misconception that being a peer did not mean being similar, nor trying to feign similarity. In fact, it is inappropriate to try and match a peer to a person based on shared diagnosis as this would be to misunderstand how peers' function. Arbitrary pairings based on perceived surface-level similarities, such as diagnosis or sociocultural characteristics, is to take an overly reductionist approach that restricts individuals to one aspect of identity and fails to recognise them as a complex human being. The peer identity is to be authentic to one's own identity and experience, it is not a deficit identity rooted in trauma. This allows them to relate so genuinely to the CYPs experience, compared to adults or clinicians, and gave them the perception of 'being human' rather than inauthentic.

'Be There With Them' – CYP Peers are Seen as 'Cultural Insiders' Whereas Adults/Clinicians are Seen as 'Cultural Outsiders'

Through showing they 'have been' where the CYP being supported is, a CYP peer establishes themselves as a 'cultural insider'. To be an 'insider' is to be able to understand and fluidly navigate the cultural spaces and norms of a group. This typically comes from being a native, i.e., a default member by one's own sociocultural or geographic status, but 'outsiders' can progress to 'insiders' if they can demonstrate sufficient cultural competence. The topic of 'outsider' and 'insider' is nuanced (for deeper understanding, see Merriam et al., 2010), but a basic understanding might be that insiders share a culture and mutual understanding of one another, whereas an outsider[5] may be perceived by an 'insider' as a threat and distrusted (Merriam et al., 2010; Naeeke et al., 2012). Such relational dynamics do not always occur, and there can be advantages when studying an 'insider' culture as an 'outsider' (Merriam et al, 2010; Naaeke et al., 2012), but when building trusting relationships, as is the aim of peer work, insider-to-insider relationships do have an advantage here. For CYP peers, they are natives to the culture, in that they share close proximity in age to CYP, especially in contrast to adult clinicians. However, to share native status is not to say that one remains an insider, and to be working in MHS can lead to being perceived as a clinician, which would revoke the insider status (a concept explored by Merriam et al., 2010). That is to say age is not what builds connections between CYP and CYP peers, but is perhaps best described as a necessary precursor, i.e., through being closer in age, CYP peers are eligible for membership within this cultural community if they can prove this cultural understanding.

CYP peers share the culture of CYP accessing services through their lived experience of being a child and young person, as well as having lived with, or continuing to live with, mental health challenges. In the study, a key part of this experience was an understanding of what it is like to be treated insincerely or disempowered by adults. CYP frequently inhabit places where they are positioned as the disempowered party with the least decision-making capacity, e.g., schools and at home, with their voices tokenised or worse, ignored completely, if they do not align with the dominant party. This can be seen in healthcare where CYP are patronised, coerced, berated, invalidated, gaslit or threatened with in-patient stays/service discharge if they do not agree with the practitioner.[6] It is easy to reject this critique as hyperbolic, but it reflects the realities of many CYP accessing services. It is not to say that these experiences are universal, but to dismiss such examples at face-value would only support CYPs' perceived insincerity of adult-provided/clinical care – the idea adults/clinicians are 'paid to be there' and do not understand young people [finding from the study]. One young person described that clinicians have

> a very adult perspective and saying well, you know, "it gets better", and you're like yeah but, you know, you're older than me now and how do you know? And have you ever been in CAMHS?
>
> Research Participant

This reveals a clear barrier to working with adult clinicians in services – one which CYP peers are best placed to overcome. CYP peers can be seen to bring a non-judgemental, validating approach that listens to and understands CYP concerns, while also allowing them to more authentically empathise with these difficulties. Through doing so, CYP peers are creating space for stories of experience that showcase divergent realities from the presumed norm. There is room to speak these and to listen to these in a reciprocal fashion, whereby both parties can tell and listen to one another's stories, and in doing so they can unveil and validate the hidden realities experienced by disempowered communities (Bell et al., (2008) defines these as 'concealed stories'). Within the study, peers referred to this as a co-created language of recovery shared by the CYP and the peer – two people who can trust one another enough to be vulnerable and share their experiences without fear of being coddled or criticised. Utilising their lived experience to build connections grants an insider status to CYP peers which fosters more trusting relationships that facilitate greater autonomy.

'A Stepping Stone' – CYP Peers Function as a 'Bridge' Between CYP and Adult, and Non-clinical and Clinical

There is a duality of liminality to the CYP peer role: they bridge the gap between the realms of non-clinical and clinical and between CYP and adults. Research has long noted the 'liminal position' (Watson, 2017, p.8) of peer support work, whereby a peer can navigate the spaces of clinical and non-clinical to facilitate better communication and support. This is supported by a research participant, who noted:

I'd describe it as being the bridge, um, between young people and services. It's about making sure young people have a voice.

Research Participant

This remains true for CYP peers, but another dimension was generated from the study – the CYP-to-adult dynamic. In a similar vein to other peer work, instead of requiring the CYP to immediately function within the confines of clinical working, the CYP peer can 'meet them at a place where [the child or young person] is comfortable' [study finding], i.e., they use the perspective of the CYP as the starting point. The CYP peer can work with the CYP to explore what their experiences have been, find out about their wants and interests, and use this as a guiding compass through services. They further facilitate access in their ability to debunk jargon and can build the confidence and know-how of the CYP by taking collaborative approaches to investigating services. However, what makes this approach more unique to CYP peer work is that they must also navigate the dynamic of adult to CYP, as well as the usual dynamic of non-clinical to clinical. A CYP peer understands what it is like to be dis-empowered as a young person, but also how it is to be disempowered due to lived experience of mental health challenges. This dual dynamic can be better navigated by someone who has lived experience elements of both, due to the unique nature of the experience. In this sense, CYP peer support can be seen as a culturally appropriate form of peer support.[7]

'Pay your Peers' – CYP Peers have a Culturally Transformative Role that Presupposes a Redistribution of Power

CYP-to-CYP support was explored to be a powerful and valuable act, but it requires fair payment of the CYP peer in order for the role to be ethical and validated in its contributions. One of the most heavily commented upon elements of the study was around the renumeration for the work of CYP peers. Though it was recognised that 'obviously' CYP peers should be paid[8] for their work, this call for 'pay your peers' was not an expression of desire for financial gain, per se. Instead, sufficient pay was equated with validation and respect of the CYP peer role, something that was seen as lacking due to the lower pay rate of a peer in comparison to the other mental health professional roles they work alongside.

One research participant phrased it like this:

It really is a fight to kind of be respected and kind of paid what you're due because you don't ask anyone else in that team to, say seven or eight times a day, [recall] memories from traumatic events in their life, you know.

RESEARCH PARTICIPANT

Where payment is interpreted as formal recognition for the value of a role, to pay one role (the peer role) significantly less than other roles is to assess peer work as innately less important and the time and effort of peers to be less valuable. In part, the lack of perceived value for peers was attributed to it being a lived experience role, lacking the academic/vocational expertise that valorised other mental health professional roles. However, CYP peers explained how the lived experience element of the role is actually one of the most challenging aspects, and how it can be difficult both to appropriately draw upon lived experiences of mental health as well as to listen to these experiences from the CYP they supported. Not only this, but other studies have shown that peer support work more than pays for itself, some showing that the return being almost 500% of the initial investment (Trachtenberg et al., 2013; Newton et al., 2017). With this in mind, the call for fair pay for peers is to not only use economic capital to validate the social capital of the peer role, but it is to justly recognise and reward them for the benefits they provide.

However, the importance of pay was only one layer to the multidimensional power structure surrounding CYP peer work that came about through the generation of this theme. Beyond pay, some peers expressed a complex relationship with other mental health professionals alongside whom they worked. They explained how there were clear feelings of uncertainty and discomfort held by both themselves and staff when they were new to the team. Peers spoke in a way that revealed internalised feelings of inadequacy and imposter syndrome. They believed they were not entitled to be there, which was exemplified for those who were working with the same staff members who had supported them when they had accessed services themselves. These feelings were seemingly qualified by the external factors: CYP accessing services did not understand their role at first and questioned why they were there, and the role was described as 'emerging' and that peers were having to carve out what their role was. Despite holding positions of employment, they explicitly described their relationships with the rest of the non-peer team as being '**almost** equal to them', that they were not quite deserving of the same respect.

These feelings of inadequacy and being an imposter were clearly difficult to grapple with, and some used self-deprecating humour as a way to express them, whereas others felt the need to justify the validity of the role. Not only this, but some of the peers valorised the more traditional mental health roles very highly, explaining how peers could not do their role without them. Here we can see the imposition of a hierarchy of ability and capability between peers and non-peers. It was established through initial peer anxiety and feelings of being an imposter, then reinforced by negative staff perception and reaction, and this has led to further inter-nalisation of inadequacy whereby the peers place other vocations on a pedestal and are made to question their innate worth. CYP peers present a challenge to the existing hierarchy, but, when this can be circumvented, it can be a powerful form of support for CYP to access and offers opportunities for authentic empathy and positive role modelling to those feeling alienated from other mental health support offers.

'The Question of Safety' – CYP Peers have a Difficult Role that Requires Role-specific Support

The final theme generated from the study was that CYP peers require suitable support in place to allow them to thrive in their role. Peers mentioned a variety of prerequisites that should be in place before they come into role/should be upheld while they are in role, including:

- training to work as a peer
- supervision while in role
- wellbeing support, including, but not limited to, wellbeing at work plans/safety plans etc.
- opportunities to develop peer work skills as well as other transferable skills
- 'strengths-focused infrastructure', i.e., staff and systems that uphold recovery-focused values.

These forms of support are required due to the specific challenges posed by the role: a peer works with their trauma as well as others, and they must uphold the boundary of being an empowerer/collaborator in recovery, and not made responsible for other's recoveries. Peer organisational support needs have long been written about, and specific guidance has been offered about these factors, as well as how it should be implemented (Repper, 2013b; Repper et al., 2021). In addition to these, peers also raised the importance of a sufficient gap between a CYP accessing initial support from MHS and becoming a peer. This was phrased as ensuring the recovery elements they are drawing from are sufficiently 'retrospective' and they are not having to drudge through difficulties with which they are currently grappling and working through. It was acknowledged that peers are often in a continuous position of recovery, and from this we can see that a temporal boundary of 'x number of months' between a difficulty occurring and a CYP peer being able to use this safely would be an erroneous interpretation of this message. Instead, we might consider this safety as being established based on a CYPs own feelings of readiness and capability, combined with the completion of suitable training. With the more surface level or 'semantic' (Clarke, 2018) nature of this theme, it may be dismissed as inconsequential compared to previous themes. However, the support needs underlying peer work must not be trivialised and the need to highlight these reveals how the onus of responsibility for having their own needs met can too frequently fall on a CYP peer's shoulders. This links back to how the peer role was still seen as 'emerging', with one peer explaining that when they joined, their manager 'had no idea what [the peer] role was'. Resultantly, this peer has been placed in the position whereby they must advocate for their needs to be met and are made responsible for designing their role. As a takeaway, it should be noted that there are fundamental support requirements for all CYP peers, and while it is positive that many of those in the role are aware of this, the burden of responsibility must be shared between organisation, team, and the CYP peer as an individual.

Conclusion

CYP peers work with similar values, skills, and ways of working as adult peers, but they are better placed to work with other CYP because they can do so more authentically, in a way that challenges the prevailing cultural hierarchy. Their experience of being a child and young person who lived/lives with mental health challenges, combined with their close proximity in age, presented in an honest, authentic way permits them to negotiate cultural insider status. In this sense, a case can be made to argue that CYP peer support is a form of culturally appropriate peer support. The empowerment of a group so traditionally unempowered in MHS poses challenges for the implementation of a CYP peer workforce, but the CYP-to-CYP support connection can be very powerful for those who experience it, when done correctly. In order to do so, it is important that both CYP peers and their organisations take full responsibility for creating and upholding the necessary support structures within which CYP peers can grow and thrive.

Parent/Carer Peers

While this chapter focuses on the CYP-to-CYP dimension of peer support provision, it would be remiss to not mention the role of parent/carer peers. Parents and caregivers play a fundamental role in keeping a child/young person safe and well, and in assisting the child/young person to develop the ability to self-manage their own safety and wellbeing (American Psychological Association, 2009). When a child/young person is struggling with their mental health, parent/carers are often affected by the difficulties themselves and may play a key role in supporting the child/young person through their recovery journey (Day et al., 2012; The Charlie Waller Trust, 2022). As such, considering the child/young person within the context of their support structures and how these all function and interplay is paramount for the child/young person's wellbeing, as well as all others involved. Parent/carer peers offer a vital avenue of support for the specific issues that parent/carers face in these situations, and it is important to understand how these two peer systems interrelate. This section will address key questions that succinctly define, differentiate, and contextualise the key elements of a parent/carer peer support worker, in order to compare and contrast parent/carer peer support to CYP peer support.

What Does a Parent/Carer Peer Do?

No matter the context, all peer work shares the same fundamental tenets (see 'What Does a Peer Support Worker Do?'). A peer draws upon lived experiences to connect with other individuals, so as to support them with the difficulties they are facing. This work is united in the shared principles that underpin it – values that seek to empower and understand someone through their own perspective. In this sense, a parent/carer peer is like any other peer. They have lived experience of supporting a child/young person with mental health challenges, and they draw upon this in a principled manner to support other parent/carers who are struggling.

However, peer support work can have a variety of different contexts, and this is where it differs: in its application. Peer support work can exist in almost any setting where there are communities of people united in an element of experience, as with these come specific difficulties. Some examples of peer support work settings are: mental health peers, physical health peers, neurodiverse peers, culturally appropriate peers, e.g., people of colour, LGBTQ+ people etc., CYP peers, parent/carer peers – the list goes on (Mind, 2019). A parent/carer peer will draw upon their peer principles and skills and then apply this in a way that is most appropriate for their context. This can influence anything and everything, from the way they build relationships, to the language they use, to the skills and tools that they draw upon and problems they discuss. For example, a CYP peer might be acutely aware of how the CYP is disempowered and excluded from decisions in their care, whereas a parent/carer peer might focus on the stresses and difficulties that a parent/carer faces when trying to navigate the mental health system and advocate for their child.

How is this Different from 'Regular' Peer Support Settings?

In a 'traditional' peer support setup, one individual draws upon their first-hand experience of mental health challenges so as to connect with and offer support to another individual.

In comparison, a parent/carer peer support worker uses lived experiences of supporting a child/family member who has struggled with/

continues to struggle with their mental health, so as to connect with and offer support to another parent/carer. This is to say that a parent/carer peer might live with vicarious distress and trauma, i.e., their first-hand experiences are informed by being closely involved in their child's own experiences. It is important to recognise that this form of lived experience is no less valid than experiencing something first-hand. From my experience training parent/carer peers, there can be initial feelings of imposter syndrome when entering this peer space as they can feel like they are telling someone else's story. What needs to be stressed is that a parent/carer peer is not telling the story of their child's distress, **they are telling their story of how this experience has impacted them and their family** (The Charlie Waller Trust, 2022).

Why Are They Needed?

Not only do parent/carers have a CYP with mental health challenges to support, but they often face difficulties with their own (Parenting Research Centre, 2016; Griffin, 2022). Supporting a child with mental health struggles and/or special needs can be an isolating and alienating experience, which, in turn, can lead to parents/carers developing long-standing mental health conditions (Parenting Research Centre, 2016; The Charlie Waller Trust, 2022; Griffin, 2022). Parent/carer peers can connect with parents and carers, and relate to their experiences (The Charlie Waller Trust, 2022). Not only this, but they can help them to navigate services to support their child, as well as other services to support with the parent/carer's own wellbeing (Parenting Research Centre, 2016; The Charlie Waller Trust, 2022). These peer relationships have been shown to be beneficial to parent/carer wellbeing as well as helping parents to feel more capable in supporting their children (Day et al., 2012; Parenting Research Centre, 2016). Furthermore, the service is more accessible as it helps to circumvent the stigma that parent/carers can face when supporting a child/young person with mental health difficulties. By having support offered by those who have been where someone else has been, it offers a non-judgemental space where the peers and those accessing services can feel as true equals (Parenting Research Centre, 2016; The Charlie Waller Trust, 2022).

Conclusion

Parent/carer peers offer a crucial form of support that benefits not only the parent/carers accessing services, but the entire family (Day et al., 2012; Parenting Research Centre, 2016; The Charlie Waller Trust, 2022). They are peers with lived experience in their own right and can offer the same benefits as other peers, as well as additional benefits to address the specific challenges of being a parent/carer (ibid). This means they can nicely complement the work of CYP peer support work and help to build a wrap-around system of support for family/caregiving units. With the limitations of this chapter, it is not possible on this occasion to explore this topic further. However, in a similar vein to CYP peer support, there is much scope for further research and discussion of parent/carer peer support in greater depth, so as to add much needed depth and breadth to our understanding of the benefits, challenges, and mechanisms of this phenomenon.

Where Next?

As peer support becomes more universally known and well-established, we have the chance to pause and reflect: how might this movement continue to evolve? This chapter has posited a case not just for peer support and CYP-to-CYP peer support, but for the need to reimagine what MHS could be. Peer support workers serve an important role in this transformational process as their ethos and ways of working challenge the long-established patriarchal norms and epistemologies underpinning MHS. It brings into question the ways in which we conceptualise wellness and recovery, and the roles we prescribe to those living with mental health challenges (Mead et al., 2001). To be truly self-defined and self-determined, recovery requires individuals to possess real and meaningful decision-making power, and the permission to refuse, deny, and disagree. While these might be core elements to person-centred care, there is still hesitation to fully trust and listen to the wants and needs of CYP (see 'Pay your peers' theme). As expressed by the research participants, 'there's something really powerful about young people supporting young people' and 'communities hold the solution to their own problems', so where are all the opportunities for CYP to be empowered to do so? CYP peer support can provide culturally appropriate peer support that does just this. It recentres the care and support to the CYP culture and worldview, and in doing so it changes the narrative from 'How can we fix CYP and their problems?' to 'What can we offer to CYP that can enable them to support themselves?'. Here we can see where peer support and participation, in their shared goal to provide a platform for lived experience to be used to create services that better suit and respect those who access them, might overlap in their efforts. For example, what would peer-support provision look like if it were CYP initiated – shared decisions at the top of Hart's (1992) Ladder of CYPs participation? This would be a peer support service that was designed by CYP, based on their expertise of what works best, so as to meet the wants and needs of the local demographic. It is innately centred in the worldview of CYP, which would be reflected in its methodologies and teloses, i.e., it would function in ways that are preferred and work best for CYP while aspiring to the goals decided by CYP. Creating a more synergistic relationship between peer support and participation can help to generate greater momentum behind this movement for CYP-focused service transformation. By redesigning our ideas of 'expert' and what support looks like, we can welcome greater authenticity within servicers, not just for CYP, but for all marginalised communities. The future of peer support is one of liberation and inclusion within MHS, and it starts by treating **everyone** as an expert in their recovery journey.

Notes

1 This is further explored in the research undertaken for this chapter, but is exemplified in a comment by a research participant, "I was terrible for this as a teenager: I didn't think staff were human" – Research Participant.
2 In this context, 'lived experience' is used to denominate experiences of mental health struggles and service access and navigation. In comparison, 'life experience' refers to common human experiences, such as relationships, loss of job/role in society, bereavement/grief etc. Dr Julie Repper delineates between the two categories as 'mental health problems' or not (Nationell Samverkan för Psykisk Hälsa, 2016).
3 There is great diversity in the naming of roles in participation, but for simplicity 'participant' shall be used as a catch-all term.
4 I choose to say emerging as the two lack the same universal recognition and infrastructure as other areas of mental health.
5 It must be noted that 'insiders' are typically from marginalised and disempowered cultures, whereas outsiders are typically from the dominant grouping. This is because subcultures must be able to navigate the mainstream in order to survive, whereas the mainstream have the choice to take an interest in subculture (Brake, 2003).
6 Based on study findings and my lived experience, as well as many CYP known to me, who have chosen to remain anonymous.
7 Culturally-appropriate peer support requires the individuals share the two experiential/demographic commonalities, rather than one, as is typical in peer support. For CYP peers these connections stem from their mental health experiences and a shared sociocultural community of age, i.e., being a child or young person.
8 Renumeration for work is far too often overlooked or justified through alternative arrangements, and this has been a common theme throughout my time as a consultant for CYPs mental health work when discussing how to get CYP involved.

References

American Psychological Association. (2009). Parents and caregivers are essential to children's health development. Available at: https://www.apa.org/pi/families/resources/parents-caregivers (Accessed: 18 November 2022).
Badenoch, B. (2017) *The heart of trauma: Healing the embodied brain in the context of relationships* (Norton Series on Interpersonal Neurobiology). WW Norton & Company.

Bell, L. A., Roberts, R. A., Irani, K. and Murphy, B. (2008) The storytelling project curriculum: Learning about race and racism through storytelling and the arts. Available at: http://www.columbia.edu/itc/barnard/education/stp/stp_curriculum.pdf (Accessed: 17 September 2022).

Brake, M. (2003) *Comparative youth culture: The sociology of youth cultures and youth subcultures in America, Britain and Canada.* London and New York: Routledge Taylor and Francis.

Braun, V. and Clarke, V. (2019) Reflecting on reflexive thematic analysis. *Qualitative Research in Sport, Exercise and Health* 11(4) pp. 589–597. https://doi.org/10.1080/2159676X.2019.1628806.

Braun, V. and Clarke, V. (2013) *Successful qualitative research.* London: Sage Publications.

Braun, V. and Clarke, V. (2006) Using thematic analysis in psychology. *Qualitative Research in Psychology* 3(2), pp. 77–101. https://doi.org/10.1191/1478088706qp063oa.

Brown, B. (2010) The power of vulnerability. Available at: https://www.ted.com/talks/brene_brown_the_power_of_vulnerability (Accessed: 3 July 2022).

Cambridge English Dictionary. (2022) Principle. In: *Cambridge English dictionary* [online]. Cambridge: Cambridge. http://dictionary.cambridge.org/dictionary/english/principle.

Clarke, V. (2018) Thematic analysis – an introduction. Available at: https://www.youtube.com/watch?v=5zFcC10vOVY (Accessed: 5 August 2022).

Davidson, L., Bellamy, C., Guy, K. and Miller, R. (2013) Peer support among persons with severe mental illnesses: A review of evidence and experience. *World Psychiatry* 11 (2), pp. 123–128. doi:10.1016/j.wpsyc.2012.05.009.

Day, C. (2008) Children's and young people's involvement and participation in mental health care. *Children and Adolescent Mental Health* 13 (1), pp. 2–8.

Day, C., Michelson, D., Thomson, S., Penney, C. and Draper, L. (2012). Evaluation of a peer led parenting intervention for disruptive behaviour problems in children: Community based randomised controlled trial. *BMJ* 344 (7849). doi:10.1136/bmj.e1107.

Deci, E. (2012) Promoting motivation, health, and excellence. Available at: https://tedxflourcity.com/?q=speaker/2012/ed-deci (Accessed: 7 July 2022).

Deegan, P. (1988) Recovery: The lived experience of rehabilitation. *Psychosocial Rehabilitation Journal* 11 (4), pp. 11–19.

Faulkner, A. and Kalathil, K. (2012) *The freedom to be, the chance to dream: Preserving user-led peer support in mental health.* London: Together.

Fortuna, K L., Solomon, P., and Rivera, J. (2022) An update of peer support/peer provided services underlying processes, benefits, and critical ingredients. *Psychiatric Quarterly*, 93 (1), pp. 571–586.

Griffin, J. (2022) Loneliness and parent carer mental health. Available at: https://cerebra.org.uk/research/loneliness-and-parent-carer-mental-health/ (Accessed 18 November 2022).

Hart, R. A. (1992) Children's participation: From tokenism to citizenship. *UNICEF International Child Development Centre* (4). Florence: Innocenti essays.

Health Education England. (2020) The Competence Framework for Mental Health Peer Support Workers. Part 1: Supporting document. Available at: https://www.

hee.nhs.uk/sites/default/files/documents/The%20Competence%20Framework%20fo
r%20MH%20PSWs%20-%20Part%201%20-%20Supporting%20document_0.pdf
(Accessed 30 July 2022).

Mead, S. (2014) *Intentional peer support: An alternative approach.* West Chester-
field: Intentional Peer Support.

Mead, S. and MacNeil, C. (2017) Peer support: What makes it unique? Available at:
https://docs.google.com/document/d/1csIJZuuh2r6h_R6U6IilRHrmszKg1wi9KtL
BbhttuPs/edit (Accessed: 7 July 2022).

Mead, S. and Filson, B. (2017) Mutuality and shared power as an alternative to
coercion and force. *Mental Health Social Inclusion*, 21 (3), pp. 144–152.
doi:10.1108/MHSI-03-2017-0011.

Mead, S., Hilton, D., and Curtis, L. (2001) Peer support: A theoretical perspective.
Psychiatric Rehabilitation Journal, 25 (2), pp. 134–141.

Merriam, S. B., Johnson-Bailey, J., Lee, M-K., Kee, Y., Ntseane, G., and Maza-
nah, M. (2010) Power and positionality: Negotiating insider/outsider status
within and across cultures, *International Journal of Lifelong Education*, 20 (5),
pp. 405–416.

Mind. (2019) Peer support. Available at: https://www.mind.org.uk/information-
support/drugs-and-treatments/peer-support/about-peer-support/ (Accessed 18
November 2022).

Naaeke, A., Kurylo, A., Grabowski, M., Linton, D. and Radford, M. L. (2012)
Insider and Outsider Perspective in Ethnographic Research. *Proceedings of the
New York State Communication Association*, 2010 (9), pp. 152–160.

Nationell Samverkan för Psykisk Hälsa. (2016) Föreläsning av professor Julie
Repper om peer support. Available at: https://www.youtube.com/watch?v=ztSY
Dum3y1E.

Newton, A., Womer, J., and Whatmough, S. (2017) *Peer support in accommoda-
tion based support services: A social return on investment.* London: Together for
Mental Wellbeing.

Park, Y. S., Konge, L., and Artino, A. R. Jr.. (2020). The positivism paradigm of
research. *Academic Medicine* 95(5), pp. 690–694. https://doi.org/10.1097/ACM.
0000000000003093.

Parenting Research Centre. (2016) Evidence summary: Peer support interventions for
parents. Available at: https://www.parentingrc.org.au/wp-content/uploads/2018/01/
EvidenceSummary_PeerSupport_Jul2016.pdf (Accessed: 18 November 2022).

Perkins, R., Repper, J. (2022) The Value and Use of Personal Experience in
Mental Health Practice. *ImROC Briefing Paper 20*. ImROC.

Repper, J. (2013a) *Peer support workers: Theory and practice.* London: Centre for
Mental Health.

Repper, J. (2013b) *Peer support workers: A practical guide to implementation.*
London: Centre for Mental Health.

Repper, J. and Carter, T., (2011) A review of the literature on peer support in
mental health services. *Journal of Mental Health*, 20 (4), pp. 392–411.

Repper, J., Walker, L., Skinner, S., and Ball, M. (2021) *Preparing organisations for
peer support: Creating a culture and context in which peer support workers
thrive.* London: Centre for Mental Health.

Repper, J. and Watson, E. (2012) A year of peer support in Nottingham: The peer
support workers and their work with individuals. *The Journal of Mental Health*

Training, Education and Practice 7 (2), pp. 79–84. doi:10.1108/17556221211236475.

Scott, A. (2011) Authenticity work: Mutuality and boundaries in peer support. *Society and Mental Health* 1(3), pp. 173–184. doi:10.1177/2156869311431101.

The Charlie Waller Trust. (2022) Parent carer peer support. Available at: https://charliewaller.org/parent-carer-peer-support/ (Accessed 18 November 2022).

Trachtenberg, M., Parsonage, M., Shepherd, G., and Boardman, J. (2013) Peer support in mental health care: Is it good value for money? Available at: https://www.centreformentalhealth.org.uk/sites/default/files/2018-09/peer_support_value_for_money_2013.pdf (Accessed 3 October 2022).

Watson, E. (2017) The mechanisms underpinning peer support: a literature review. *Journal of Mental Health*. https://doi.org/10.1080/09638237.2017.1417559.

Chapter 14

Why participation requires systemic culture change and how we get there

Hannah Sharp (She/Her)

Introduction: The Need for Systemic Culture Change

From the text so far, it is evident that good participation is founded in the behaviour of individuals who facilitate it. At the micro-level, the individual practitioner must change the way they work to include participation as a driving part of their practice. For example, by actively trying to involve the patient in shared decision-making. At the meso-level, service managers must seek out and choose to value the voices of patients. At the macro-level, national teams must choose to facilitate the involvement of patients and carers in all that they do. Improving participation cannot be achieved without changing behaviour.

'Behaviour' itself is not a stand-alone concept. It is shaped by attitudes and values. While the relationship between attitudes and behaviour cannot be considered directly correlated, it is the modern thought that the latter is at least shaped by the former (Manstead, 1996). Attitudes rest upon the knowledge, experiences, beliefs, and assumptions individuals have/make about the world (Regan and Fazio, 1977). It therefore makes sense to conclude that to change behaviour requires increasing the knowledge held by an individual and shaping their experience and assumptions in order to change their attitudes and resulting behaviour.

This change, however, needs to be system-wide because of the structures needed to support good participation. Without the proper structures in place to take and act upon patient feedback, tokenism can occur (as discussed in Chapter 3) and if different therapeutic options are not accessible for a patient, they cannot make choice and have a say in their own care. To enable micro-level participation, the clinician must have support from the meso- and macro-levels to facilitate choice. At the meso-level, national policy must enable flexibility in service delivery to allow services to act on feedback and clinicians must support the collection of this feedback. At the macro-level, services must contribute to national outcome measures and present opportunities to young people for involvement on this scale. Participation doesn't happen on isolated occasions within a system, it is a consistent flow of communication and action throughout all parties within that system.

DOI: 10.4324/9781003288800-14

This forces us to consider behaviour change on a larger scale. To change the behaviour of all those within a system requires a consideration of the context the system provides. This is where the concept of 'organisational culture' becomes important. Within a system, some of the knowledge, beliefs and attitudes that influence behaviour are shared. It would be unfair to suggest they are entirely shared, there is naturally still room for individual autonomy of thought otherwise new ideas and trailblazers of best practice surrounding participation would not emerge. It would also, however, be naïve to suggest that individuals are not influenced by the beliefs and behaviours of those around them. This is a widely accepted fact in social psychology (Bar-Tal, 2000). This way of thinking is what shapes Mannion and Davies' (Mannion and Davies, 2018) model of organisational culture, which is presented in Figure 14.1 below.

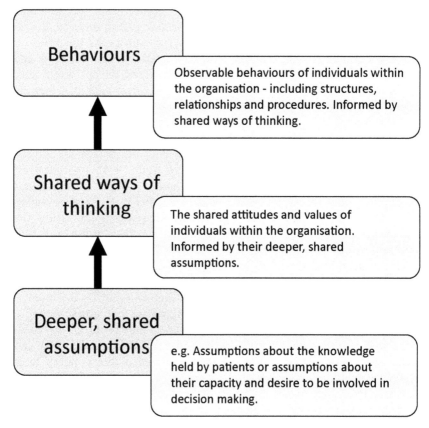

Figure 14.1 An illustration of Mannion and Davies' (2018) conception of organisational culture within healthcare organisations

On this basis, it makes sense that in order to change collective behaviour relating to participation on a systemic level, we need systemic culture change. But how do we do this? How do we change assumptions, knowledge, and attitudes on such a large scale? It is here I wish to turn to an example of where we have done this before, and we've done it before relating to participation in Children and Young People's Mental Health (CYPMH).

Introducing Children and Young People's Improving Access to Psychological Therapies (CYP-IAPT)

In 2011, Child and Adolescent Mental Health Services (CAMHS) was inaccessible. It faced rising rates of referrals resulting in lengthy waiting lists and a high acuity threshold for access. There was a high frequency of missed appointments, transition between different parts of CAMHS was poor and outcomes were not routinely scrutinised (Department of Health, 2011a; Fonagy et al., 2017; Shafran et al., 2014). In a context of rising levels of poor child and adolescent mental health, and increasing social and political interest in the area (Fonagy et al., 2016), systemic change in CAMHS was recognised by the Department of Health as a vital next step in their journey to improve the mental health of the nation (Department of Health, 2011b, 2011a).

Children and Young People (CYP), parents, and carers were not routinely consulted for their opinions on services or involved in key decisions about their care (Fonagy et al., 2017). Feedback was broadly not being acted upon, though there were some examples of positive change. Their feedback was also being given to services via research projects rather than it being entrenched in the workings of the service (Worrall-Davies, 2008). A limited focus on participation meant that other competing interests took precedent for example, reducing waiting lists (Worrall-Davies, 2008). This was particularly the case for participation at the meso-level (Day, 2008).

Concerns remained about the capacity of CYP to be involved. Providing accessible information to CYP to facilitate their participation was an ongoing debate surrounding issues such as the format it should take or how complex the content could be. Tools to facilitate participation in CAMHS were in early stages of development, had not yet been evaluated and were still viewed as 'novel' (Day, 2008). There were also concerns that providing certain information to CYP could be detrimental to their care (Day, 2008; Pollock et al., 2004). However, participation in CAMHS was concretely on the policy agenda.

CYP-IAPT aimed to achieve transformation in CAMHS via a number of key changes. These can be summarised as: an increased use of evidence-based therapies (EBTs), consistent use of routine outcome measures (ROMs) and greater participation (Department of Health, 2011a; Edbrooke-Childs et al., 2015; Ludlow et al., 2020a; Shafran et al., 2014).

It took place in, what was at the time, tier 2 and 3 community CAMHS, reflecting the growing emphasis on deinstitutionalisation and 'care in the community' (Hadland and Ehresmann, 2016; The Health Foundation and The King's Fund, 2015). Services were invited to apply to become part of a system of 'collaboratives'. These collaboratives involved a partnership between individual services, the voluntary sector, and higher education institutions (HEIs). The HEIs were responsible for providing the support and training of staff based upon a 'national CYP-IAPT curriculum' (NHS England, 2011) which included training frontline staff on EBTs and ROMs (Department of Health, 2011c). Part of the application process for these collaboratives was the requirement for services to establish these partnerships and demonstrate their capacity to implement the programme. This included appropriate 'buy-in' from senior management, evidence that the HEIs they intended to partner with had the ability to provide their staff with training, evidence that they were able to comply with outcomes monitoring, and a demonstration of how they intended to deliver the parts of the programme requiring local flexibility – for example, participation (Department of Health, 2011c).

Early documentation on the project states that it was developed in partnership with CYP, and thus had participation at its core (Department of Health, 2011d; Fonagy and Clark, 2015; NHS England, 2012). But it is impossible, from the literature alone, to determine the quality of that partnership. With this phase of the project occurring 10 years ago at the time of writing, it is also unlikely that it can be determined via a practical research approach effectively.

Participation was integrated throughout all three core components of the programme (EBTs, ROMs, and participation) despite having its own distinct component. CYP were involved in the training of staff via the collaboratives, and often this included training practitioners on EBTs (Shafran et al., 2014, p. 160). They were also involved in the development and selection of appropriate ROMs (Department of Health, 2011a). ROMs also facilitated participation at the micro-level, particularly via the use of goal-based outcomes (GBOs), which allowed the CYP to steer their individual treatment towards their own goals. GBOs were therefore a key facilitator for shared decision-making (SDM). The 'Session rating scale' ROM also provided an opportunity for patients to feed back into service improvement and thus be involved in meso-level participation (Child Outcomes Research Consortium, n.d.; Edbrooke-Childs et al., 2015; Hall et al., 2013; Law et al., 2014). Finally, the participation component of the programme covered all aspects of participation not covered by the other components and reinforced their partial purposes for SDM and service development via other means such as other training as part of the learning collaboratives.

CYP-IAPT ceased as a standalone project in 2015 and was integrated into a broader CAMHS transformation strategy as part of delivering on the 'Future in Mind' report (Department of Health, 2015). This new strategy saw a significant shift in focus from workforce development to workforce and service expansion (Ludlow et al., 2020b). It sought to encompass more services, such as schools, to provide CYP with a broader package of care (Hadland and Ehresmann, 2016; Mcdougall, 2016). There was less of a focus on participation than in CYP-IAPT when it was a standalone programme and, as I shall discuss later in the chapter, significant progress in participation occurred over the period from 2011–2015. Consequently, I will be focusing on this timeframe.

CYP-IAPT: The Challenges of Implementing Patient Participation

CYP-IAPT faced the ultimate challenge discussed so far in this book, changing the attitudes and behaviours of those involved in CAMHS. At the micro-level, the individual practitioner must change the way they work to include participation as a driving part of their practice. Unlike other changes, such as introducing a new procedure, participation cannot just be routinised (Collins et al., 2007). Therefore, though not outwardly expressed by CYP-IAPT, it was stimulating systemic culture change, which must be the main means by which it improved participation (Anderson and Sharp, 2020). To create change like this on a national scale throughout all layers of the CAMHS system involves thousands of individuals. This is a significant undertaking.

I do wish to make an important aside note here. Despite the emphasis this text places on attitude change as the core way to develop participation, routinisation can help and did within CYP-IAPT. The use of ROMs to facilitate participation at the micro-level created a means of continuous feedback and monitoring for the national project team. Learning from other failed transformation programmes, particularly those of Stark County and Fort Bragg (Andrade et al., 2000; Bickman et al., 1997), CYP-IAPT was informed by implementation science principles from its conception (Fonagy and Clark, 2015; Shafran et al., 2014). Not only did this allow the national team to receive feedback on the project, but it also made opportunities for participation at the micro-level mandatory. I have termed these 'opportunities' because with routinisation comes the risk for tokenism. However, by presenting these opportunities practitioners are reminded consistently of their obligation to involve the patient in their care. Although ultimately, they must hold an attitude that includes wanting to use ROMs meaningfully. You cannot 'routinise' an attitude.

The main purpose of the collaborative system was to facilitate a quality improvement (QI) approach that enabled services to gradually introduce participation in a way that suited their service whilst still fitting within the national project guidelines (Burn et al., 2020). This flexibility helps to reduce the chance of an implementation gap because professionals are able to target their engagement in participation in a way that supports their practice, making it appear more meaningful to them and improving their attitudes towards it (Tummers and Bekkers, 2014). The system also provided the opportunity to train staff on what participation is. It also presented the chance to address misconceptions surrounding CYP-IAPT concerns that the real purpose of ROMs was performance management. These were common barriers faced throughout the implementation of the programme (Burn et al., 2020; Taylor, 2016). Furthermore, as time went on and staff had more opportunity to engage with training and the rest of the collaborative system, this scepticism decreased and simultaneously the programme's implementation improved (Edbrooke-Childs et al., 2015; Fonagy, 2014). Thus, once again, attitudes towards participation and ROMs were vital to progress.

Another key barrier to implementation was a lack of resources. Complexities in funding mean that we cannot accurately determine how much is spent on CAMHS. But there are strong indications and a consensus that it was, and still is, chronically underfunded (Baldwin, 2016; Dormon, 2015; Frith, 2016). Underfunded services often lack the infrastructure needed for technological development – such as the online systems used to collect ROMs data and submit them to national databases (Wolpert et al., 2011). This makes changes like the implementation of ROMs more challenging and time consuming. A lack of funding also impacts on staffing levels, with workforce shortages being a common report across CAMHS (though it is important to note that this is often also due to other reasons such as the general lack of trained mental health nurses in the workforce) (British Medical Association, 2019). This makes the training burden even more impactful as a loss of staff to training cannot be 'picked up' by other team members. In addition, a lack of resources makes acting on patient feedback more challenging. Not acting on patient feedback is not meaningful participation (Arnstein, 1969).

While a lack of resources may not seem to be related to attitude and culture change at first consideration, it is embroiled in the culture of service management and the NHS commissioning system. Limited funding must go where the priorities lie. This inevitably involves value judgements (Towse et al., 2002). Therefore, for participation to get more funding requires it to have greater value in the eyes of commissioners and management.

I have placed particular emphasis on the use of ROMs in the programme as they are an important demonstration of participation at the micro-level. In addition, their effective implementation has consequences at the meso-level too. There are however plenty examples of participation at the meso- and macro-levels which are even more embedded in organisational culture because they cannot be routinised in the same way. At the meso-level, participation groups and the involvement of patients in commissioning require the voice of the patient to be listened to and valued by the staff they are working alongside to avoid the trap of tokenism. The same principles apply at the macro-level with the involvement of patients in national governance and policymaking (Anderson and Sharp, 2020). Even at the micro-level, ROMs are not the only occasion of SDM. Practitioners must constantly engage in dialogue with the patients about their needs and desires to tailor their sessions beyond just goals or a rating of the session (Elwyn et al., 2012).

This discussion has addressed just some of the challenges to implementing effective participation which were identified and targeted by CYP-IAPT. Others include change fatigue, constraints on organisational change, and concerns surrounding the desire and capability of CYP to be involved in participation (Anderson and Sharp, 2020; Burn et al., 2020; Hamer, 2014; Taylor, 2016). I believe that these issues, amongst others, are either more obviously founded in culture, attitude, value, and behaviour change, or are explained by this discussion above.

Evaluating the Success of CYP-IAPT

To justify this focus on CYP-IAPT as the core example of how we create systemic culture change in CYPMH services requires an evaluation of its success. Evaluating the success of CYP-IAPT is made particularly challenging by the lack of outcomes data for the initiative. Data collected by the Child Outcomes Research Consortium (CORC), which was tasked with analysing ROMs data had a return rate of less than 25% for second scores meaning that no reliable outcomes data was collected (Timimi, 2015). This means that to evaluate the success of CYP-IAPT, evidence needs to be collected from other sources than those which were intended.

A rapid internal audit of the programme took place in 2015, which produced limited data. Two reports were produced. The first was specific to CYP and produced by the organisation 'GIFT' (Great Involvement Future Thinking) who led the patient participation element of the programme (GIFT, 2015). The second was produced by CORC (Edbrooke-Childs et al., 2015) and also included data directly from CYP. The GIFT report interviewed and surveyed 45 CYP: 35 current service users and 10 pre-CYP-IAPT service users. This is the only data available, which directly compares experiences of participation before and after CYP-IAPT. The CORC report, on the other hand, surveyed 6,803 current service users. Despite a significant difference in sample size, their findings were broadly the same. Some of the most notable statistics can be found below:

The GIFT report (2015):

- 33% of patients felt they were given enough information to aid choice about their treatments, compared with 20% who had contact with the service prior to CYP-IAPT,
- 50% said they could participate in setting goals versus 50% pre-CYP-IAPT,
- 42% knew about the complaints process compared with 40% pre-CYP-IAPT. But only 32% felt it was CYP appropriate, a fall from 50% pre-CYP-IAPT. Though the report highlights this could be explained by a high number of 'I don't know' responses,
- Fewer current patients were involved in staff training and recruitment, but this is also explained by a tendency of services to involve past service users in this work (GIFT, 2015). For the past service users consulted responses were notably high with 60–85% of CYP reporting involvement,
- 52% of current patients met with senior managers versus 33% of past service users, and 75% of current patients felt managers acted on their feedback versus 65% pre-CYP-IAPT,
- 68% of patients knew there was a participation group versus 70% pre-CYP-IAPT. Though this could be explained by 'I don't know' responses and the tendency to involve past service users,
- 48% identified changes resulting from participation vs 57% pre-CYP-IAPT. But this could also be explained by 'I don't know' responses.

The CORC report (Edbrooke-Childs et al., 2015):

- 50% of patients reported being involved in goal setting as part of their treatment,
- 61% said there was a regular participation group. Note: services may have a participation group which a patient was unaware of and thus answered 'no' to this question,
- 45% could identify change resulting from participation,
- 41% reported they were involved in the delivery of staff training and 25% said they had a say in the content of training,
- 47% of patients met with senior managers and of those, 61% felt listened to and 71% thought management acted on their views,
- Overall, 83% of patients felt they were able to give feedback about their service.

The CORC report also approached clinicians for their feedback and they reported similar, or marginally higher, rates of success. Some of the notable statistics are below:

- 84% of clinicians reported that patients were encouraged to participate in their treatment and reviews,
- 40% said patients were invited to management meetings,
- 65% reported changes to the service environment based on patient feedback,
- 61% of clinicians reported changes to the delivery of care,
- 43% said there were changes to the choice of therapy,
- 40% identified changes to staff training and 55% reported changes to recruitment involving patients.

There are important limitations to both sets of data. The obvious limitation with the GIFT report is the small sample size. While the CORC report had a larger sample size, it is still a small percentage of CAMHS patients – though the sample was more diverse and fairly representative of the CAMHS patient demographic (Edbrooke-Childs et al., 2015). The CORC report also had a further notable limitation. Its inclusion criteria selected services that were more engaged with CYP-IAPT. The impact of this selection is debatable. If we are evaluating the impact of CYP-IAPT when properly implemented, then this is acceptable and more accurate. But if it's only picking its best services, it is not a reflection of the reality of CYP-IAPT as a whole. While selected services could provide more comprehensive data for the audit, getting a full picture with limited data for other services is also valuable. Perhaps the most important limitation, however, is that the patients giving feedback on a service are naturally more likely to be the patients who know that there are opportunities to give feedback on their service. Nevertheless, both reports demonstrate at least some progress towards better participation.

As I have highlighted above, there is limited 'before and after' data available for CYP-IAPT. A qualitative exploration of examples from CYP-IAPT is more capable of providing a better picture of participation before, during, and after its delivery.

One of the most common changes made by services was the introduction or improvement of a 'patient participation group' to provide meso-level feedback on the service. While we cannot gain an understanding of how tokenistic or meaningful this participation was, we can see that there was a change towards understanding their importance via how they were used. For example, Torbay CAMHS established a patient participation group and worked with over 25 CYP over a 2-year period and report that patients were 'actively engaged' in staff recruitment and service development (Young, 2014). 5 Boroughs Partnership NHS Foundation Trust re-launched their participation group and held a stakeholder conference specifically for CYP (Woods and Parsons, 2014). Cheshire and the Wirral CAMHS also involved patients in training and recruitment (Walker et al., 2014). A final example of many possible choices is that Oxleas CAMHS set up CYP participation groups across boroughs and services to engage with more CYP (Walker et al., 2014).

At the macro-level, GIFT facilitated CYP participation on a scale not seen before in CAMHS governance, and perhaps also the rest of the NHS. Their patient advisors, who were paid for their time, attended national board meetings, co-chaired the national CYP-IAPT board, advised on national service specifications, advised policy via the Health Select Committee, and ran national conferences. They became fully integrated in the national governance of the project as time progressed and meetings became tailored to enable their meaningful participation (Anderson and Sharp, 2020; Walker et al., 2014).

At the micro-level it becomes harder to find examples because it involved individual occasions of treatment. However, it is important to remember that the introduction of GBOs themselves is micro-level participation. There are also some quotes from clinicians in reviews of the project, which indicate that CYP-IAPT played a strong role in changing the culture around participation in their organisation. For example, in the rapid internal audit (Edbrooke-Childs et al., 2015) staff reported that:

> attitudes around working more collaboratively with children and families…changed.
>
> (p.23)

> CYP were perceived to have felt a greater sense of ownership, which facilitates important discussions that might not take place otherwise.
>
> (p.24)

> Although [one clinician's] service already used the Goal Based Outcome (GBO) measure before CYP IAPT, the programme had resulted in "real cultural change" in the integration of the GBO into clinical practice and the sharing of data, as opposed to a "tickboxy" approach.
>
> (p.44)

> Most interviewees reported that CYP-IAPT resulted in the increased voice of CYP "in a massive way" (p.31). They also support my earlier assertion that culture change was necessary to implement participation, as some clinicians reported finding the use of ROMs "clunky" and a "challenge". Despite this, over the course of the programme, they became "embedded" and "more fluent" within their practice.
>
> (p.44)

But there also exists evidence that CYP might not feel the same positivity towards participation, particularly GBOs (Edbrooke-Childs et al., 2015).

Though here, it is important to note that effective implementation takes time and there is evidence that CYP-IAPT caused the culture change which can then drive staff towards improving their implementation. Changes like this take time to be presented in data, which is why looking towards qualitative examples can be beneficial (Anderson and Sharp, 2020). These examples therefore show what the data does not show so clearly that strong, positive steps were taken by services to, at the very least, begin to implement CYP-IAPT's participation principles.

It is important to distill, however, whether this change would, or even could, have happened without CYP-IAPT. There was already policy momentum towards improving participation in CAMHS. If the answer to this question is 'yes', this could render CYP-IAPT a bureaucratic waste of time, which added unnecessary complexity and pressure on an already struggling CAMHS system.

There is evidence that progress towards CYP-IAPT's goals relating to participation took place externally to the programme. Services that were not part of CYP-IAPT reported changes relating to participation over the period of 2011–2015. For example, North Bristol NHS Foundation Trust (NBT) initiated their own children's community health transformation programme specifically focusing on participation, with CAMHS highlighted as one of its central focuses (Brady et al., 2020). At the beginning of their programme, NBT faced many of the same challenges that CYP-IAPT identified relating to participation such as poor support from management, a lack of staff understanding, and negative attitudes towards participation (Brady et al., 2020). Their 2015 Care Quality Commission (CQC) report demonstrates their success in changing this culture. It stated that participation was 'routinely' included in every aspect of the service and was an 'outstanding' example of participation nationally (Care Quality Commission, 2015, p. 4). It created the same change as CYP-IAPT, but was not part of the programme.

Culture change also took place beyond CYP-IAPT. For example, the Quality Network for Community CAMHS (QNCC) at the Royal College of Psychiatrists (RcPsych) acts as a network for sharing best practice and expected standards of care. QNCC demonstrates the increasing importance of participation via their rating system for standards. It describes its standards in the following terms (The Quality Network for Community CAMHS, 2013):

- 'Type 1' standards: 'failure to meet these standards would result in a significant threat to patient safety, rights or dignity and/or would breach the law',
- 'Type 2' standards: 'standards that an accredited service would be expected to meet',
- 'Type 3' standards: 'standards that an excellent service should meet or standards that are not the direct responsibility of the team'.

Between 2012 and 2015, 3 of 15 standards directly relating to participation changed from type 2 to type 1 standards and a new type 1 participation standard was introduced. Three participation standards were removed (The Quality Network for Community CAMHS, 2016, 2013).

QNCC standards go through a revision process whereby all member CAMHS work to reach a consensus on changes to the standards (The Quality Network for Community CAMHS, 2020). When all member services reach a consensus on changing a standard, this demonstrates their agreement on what quality care looks like. In addition, 25% of standards were removed between 2012 and 2015 (The Quality Network for Community CAMHS, 2016, 2013). Therefore, to only experience the net loss of two standards relating to participation shows that participation is viewed by QNCC member CAMHS as a core part of their service.

It is possible that the NBT programme and QNCC standards were influenced by CYP-IAPT. Changing cultures within CYP-IAPT services may have radiated to others via networks such as QNCC due to CYP-IAPT increasing the expected standards of care for services more broadly. There is also potential that it did not. This is a debate we are likely to never know the answer to, but alongside the other evidence I have presented there is a strong case that CYP-IAPT created strong culture change autonomously.

Returning to Organisational Culture and the Need for Quality Improvement

So what can we learn about how we continue the progress CYP-IAPT made? When we turn to how CYP-IAPT made its progress, we can identify its use of a quality improvement-based approach (Burn et al., 2020). Arasaratnam (2012, p. 257) writes that 'quality improvement can be defined as a structured analysis of a system's performance with a view to improvement'. It has numerous approaches, but can ultimately be described as a continuous cycle of learning and change (Varkey et al., 2007). There are numerous explorations of quality improvement and its methodology available, so this chapter will not seek to go into detail about its practicalities. For the sake of discussing its utility for creating culture change, thinking of it as this cycle ought to be a sufficient level of depth however, the end of this chapter will explore some of these practicalities when it comes to applying the thoughts in this chapter to practice.

Resistance to change within the NHS has become more commonplace in the wake of "excessive" change since the introduction of the internal market (Lang et al., 2004, p.4). Clinicians are sceptical towards and are disillusioned by what they see to be politically driven promises of radical change (Lang et al., 2004, p.4). A lack of clarity surrounding what participation constitutes compounds this fear and scepticism (Rowe and Shepherd, 2002; Collins et al., 2007). Clinicians want to protect their autonomy and reputation as experts and this is challenged by the introduction of greater participation, particularly at the micro-level (Salter, 2003). This resistance is what makes improved participation a particularly difficult policy to implement via QI. But it is also what makes QI the best method of implementation. Gradual culture change is necessary as implementing an entirely new policy without time for clinicians to adapt would be too challenging.

It is for these reasons, that the systemic culture change we have established is necessary to better embed the principles of better participation in CYPMH services and is best achieved via a QI approach.

A Final Note: "If CYP-IAPT Was So Successful, Why is this Book Even Necessary?"

The argument made in this chapter is not that CYP-IAPT did everything, but that it did something. It created progress towards improving participation via systemic culture change using a QI approach. But there is still progress to be made. Since the iteration of CYP-IAPT, which included a focus on participation ceased, there have been no systemic attempts to improve participation. No programmes have involved those from senior roles in NHS England all the way down to frontline practitioners. Small QI projects have taken place in individual services, but to create the pressure necessary to create large-scale change requires the involvement of those at the highest level. Without pressure being put on commissioners to fund participation via policy and participation being a national priority, for example, their limited budgets will be spent where that pressure lies.

This isn't to say local projects aren't effective. But local projects create inequality of participation. The examples of best practice shared throughout this text are trailblazing, not the norm. One of the core values of the NHS is that 'nobody is excluded, discriminated against or left behind' (Department of Health, 2021). Where we do not have a cohesive, nationally co-ordinated attempt at QI towards better participation we increase the risk of this inequality and the threat arises that people will be 'left behind'. This isn't to say a national programme alone solves this inequality, there is still differential engagement with such programmes. It does, however, decrease the likelihood that stark differences in participation will continue to arise and it ensures that where differences do arise, they are less significant and are more easily able to be resolved because the support to do so is in place.

Creating Systemic Culture Change

As discussed earlier in the chapter, creating systemic culture change is founded upon changing shared attitudes, values, and beliefs on the systemic level. There are lessons we can learn from what CYP-IAPT did well, and some of the key takeaways from this chapter are listed below for ease:

- Strong leadership and leading by example help to create a positive ethos towards participation by helping practitioners to see it as something important,
- Patience with the implementation of new projects and taking a QI approach allows clinicians to adapt and make changes at their own pace,
- Routinisation can be helpful in accelerating change, but without culture change alongside it risks tokenism,
- Educating staff helps to increase knowledge and allow professionals to develop informed opinions towards participation,
- Support is required from all levels of the system.

References

Anderson, Y., Sharp, H., 2020. *Children's Participation: Making it Happen*, in: Kick-off Participatie in de Geestelijke Gezondheidszorg, 1ste WEBINAR 7 December 2020.

Andrade, A. R., Lambert, E. W., Bickman, L., 2000. Dose effect in child psychotherapy: Outcomes associated with negligible treatment. *J. Am. Acad. Child Adolesc. Psychiatry* 39, 161–168. https://doi.org/10.1097/00004583-200002000-00014.

Arasaratnam, R., 2012. Quality improvement. *Br. J. Hosp. Med. (Lond)*. 73, 257–261. https://doi.org/10.12968/HMED.2012.73.5.257.

Arnstein, S. R., 1969. A Ladder Of Citizen Participation. *J. Am. Inst. Plann.* 35, 216–224. https://doi.org/10.1080/01944366908977225.

Baldwin, L., 2016. Changing roles in changing times, in: Mcdougall, T. (Ed.), *Children and Young People's Mental Health: Essentials for Nurses and Other Professionals*. Routledge, London.

Bar-Tal, D., 2000. Sharing beliefs in groups, in: Bar-Tal, D. (Ed.), *Shared Beliefs in a Society: Social Psychological Analysis*. SAGE Publications, Inc., California, pp. 1–6.

Bickman, L., Summerfelt, W. M. T., Firth, J. M., Douglas, S. M., 1997. The Stark County Evaluation Project: Baseline results of a randomized experiment. *Eval. Ment. Heal. Serv.* 3.

Brady, L.-M., Roberts, E., Hathway, F., Horn, L., 2020. Shifting sands: trying to embed participation in a climate of change, in: Brady, L.-M. (Ed.), *Embedding Young People's Participation in Health Services*. Bristol University Press, pp. 177–204.

British Medical Association, 2019. Measuring progress: Commitments to support and expand the mental health workforce in England. British Medical Association.

Burn, A.-M., Vainre, M., Humphrey, A., Howarth, E., 2020. Evaluating the CYP-IAPT transformation of child and adolescent mental health services in

Cambridgeshire, UK: a qualitative implementation study. *Implement. Sci. Commun.* 1, 89. https://doi.org/10.1186/s43058-020-00078-6.

Care Quality Commission, 2015. *North Bristol NHS Trust. Community health services for children, young people and families.* Quality Report.

Child Outcomes Research Consortium, n.d. *Outcome & Experience Measures* [WWW Document]. https://www.corc.uk.net/outcome-experience-measures/ (accessed 16. 3. 2021).

Collins, S., Britten, N., Ruusuvuori, J., Thompson, A., 2007. Understanding the process of patient participation, in: *Patient Participation in Health Care Consultations: Qualitative Perspectives.* Open University Press, McGraw Hill, Berkshire, pp. 3–21.

Day, C., 2008. Children's and young people's involvement and participation in mental health care. *Child Adolesc. Ment. Health* 13, 2–8. https://doi.org/10.1111/j.1475-3588.2007.00462.x.

Department of Health, 2021. The NHS constitution for England [WWW Document]. https://www.gov.uk/government/publications/the-nhs-constitution-for-england/the-nhs-constitution-for-england (accessed 26.2.2021).

Department of Health, 2015. *Future in mind - Promoting, protecting and improving our children and young people's mental health and wellbeing.* Crown Copyright.

Department of Health, 2011a. *Talking therapies: A four-year plan of action. A supporting document to No health without mental health: A cross-government mental health outcomes strategy for people of all ages.* Crown Copyright.

Department of Health, 2011b. *No Health Without Mental Health: A cross-government mental health outcomes strategy for people of all ages,* Policy.

Department of Health, 2011c. *Children and Young People's IAPT project. Applying to become a Phase One Learning Collaborative.* Crown Copyright.

Department of Health, 2011d. *No health without mental health A cross-government mental health outcomes strategy for people of all ages.* Crown Copyright.

Dormon, F., 2015. Changes in CAMHS: parity or warm words? [WWW Document]. *Heal. Found.* https://health.org.uk/blogs/changes-in-camhs-parity-or-warm-words (accessed 17. 5. 2021).

Edbrooke-Childs, J., Calderon, A., Wolpert, M., Fonagy, P., 2015. *Rapid Internal Audit National Report.* Child outcomes research consortium.

Elwyn, G., Frosch, D., Thomson, R., Joseph-Williams, N., Lloyd, A., Kinnersley, P., Cording, E., Tomson, D., Dodd, C., Rollnick, S., Edwards, A., Barry, M., 2012. Shared decision making: A model for clinical practice. *J. Gen. Intern. Med.* https://doi.org/10.1007/s11606-012-2077-6.

Fonagy, P., 2014. *Professor Peter Fonagy - CYP IAPT National Clinical Lead,* in: CYP IAPT Conference 2014.

Fonagy, P., Clark, D.M., 2015. Update on the improving access to psychological therapies programme in england: commentary on … children and young people's improving access to psychological therapies. *BJPsych Bull.* 39, 248–251. https://doi.org/10.1192/pb.bp.115.052282.

Fonagy, P., Pugh, K., O'Herlihy, A., 2017. The Children and Young People's Improving Access to Psychological Therapies (CYP IPAT) programme in England, in: Skuse, D., Bruce, H., Dowdney, L. (Eds.), *Child Psychology and Psychiatry: Frameworks for Clinical Training and Practice.* John Wiley & Sons, Ltd, pp. 429–435.

Fonagy, P., Pugh, K., O'Herlihy, A., 2016. *Embedding Future in mind in our communities*, in: CYPMH National Annual Conference 2016.

Frith, E., 2016. Progress and challenges in the transformation of children and young people's mental health care Children and Young People's Mental Health About the author.

GIFT, 2015. Rapid audit for CYP IAPT: Young people's workstream. GIFT.

Hadland, R., Ehresmann, F., 2016. Education, training and workforce development for CAMHS nurses, in: Mcdougall, T. (Ed.), *Children and Young People's Mental Health: Essentials for Nurses and Other Professionals*. Routledge, London.

Hall, C. L., Moldavsky, M., Baldwin, L., Marriott, M., Newell, K., Taylor, J., Sayal, K., Hollis, C., 2013. The use of routine outcome measures in two child and adolescent mental health services: A completed audit cycle. *BMC Psychiatry* 13, 270. https://doi.org/10.1186/1471-244X-13-270.

Hamer, H., 2014. *Transforming children's services across the Midlands and East of England: Real life experiences of implementing routine outcome measures, increasing access to psychological therapies and promoting young peoples' involvement The Midlands and East Mental Health*, in: Child and Adolescent Mental Health (CAMHS) Conference 2014, The University of Northampton, 02–04 July 2014.

Lang, S., Wainwright, C. and Sehdev, K. (2004). *A review of patient choice in the NHS*. Healthcare Management Research Group, Cranfield University.

Law, D., Miller, S., Squire, B., 2014. Session Rating Scale (SRS) and Child Session Rating Scale (CSRS), in: *Guide to Using Outcomes and Feedback Tools with Children, Young People and Families*. CORC Ltd.

Ludlow, C., Hurn, R., Lansdell, S., 2020a. A Current Review of the Children and Young People's Improving Access to Psychological Therapies (CYP IAPT) Program: Perspectives on Developing an Accessible Workforce. *Adolesc. Health. Med. Ther.* 11, 21–28. https://doi.org/10.2147/ahmt.s196492.

Ludlow, C., Hurn, R., Lansdell, S., 2020b. A Current Review of the Children and Young People's Improving Access to Psychological Therapies (CYP IAPT) Program: Perspectives on Developing an Accessible Workforce. *Adolesc. Health. Med. Ther.* 11, 21–28. https://doi.org/10.2147/ahmt.s196492.

Mannion, R., Davies, H., 2018. Understanding organisational culture for healthcare quality improvement. *BMJ* 363. https://doi.org/10.1136/bmj.k4907.

Manstead, A. S. R., 1996. Attitudes and behaviours, in: Semin, G. R., Fiedler, K. (Eds.), *Applied Social Psychology*. SAGE Publications Ltd, London, pp. 3–29.

Mcdougall, T., 2016. CAMHS transformation: Modernising therapeutic interventions and outcomes, in: Mcdougall, T. (Ed.), *Children and Young People's Mental Health: Essentials for Nurses and Other Professionals*. Routledge, London.

NHS England, 2012. Children and Young Peoples Project FAQ's [WWW Document]. iapt.nhs.uk. http://web.archive.org/web/20120123063900/http://www.iapt.nhs.uk/cyp-iapt/children-and-young-peoples-project-faqs/ (accessed 14.5. 2021).

NHS England, 2011. Children and Young People's Improving Access to Psychological Therapies Project: Draft national curriculum. NHS England.

Pollock, K., Grime, J., Baker, E., Mantala, K., 2004. Meeting the information needs of psychiatric inpatients: Staff and patient perspectives. *J. Ment. Heal.* 13, 389–401. https://doi.org/10.1080/09638230410001729834.

Regan, D. T., Fazio, R., 1977. On the consistency between attitudes and behavior: Look to the method of attitude formation. *J. Exp. Soc. Psychol.* 13, 28–45. https://doi.org/10.1016/0022-1031(77)90011-90017.

Rowe, R., Shepherd, M. 2002. Public participation in the new NHS: No closer to citizen control? *Social Policy and Administration*, 36(3), 275–290. [Online] Available at: doi:10.1111/1467-9515.00251 (accessed 16 February 2021).

Salter, B. 2003. Patients and doctors: reformulating the UK health policy community? *Social Science & Medicine*, 57, 927–936.

Shafran, R., Fonagy, P., Pugh, K., Myles, P., 2014. Transformation of Mental Health Services for Children and Young People in England, in: Beidas, R.S., Kendall, P.C. (Eds.), *Dissemination and Implementation of Evidence-Based Practices in Child and Adolescent Mental Health*. Oxford University Press, pp. 158–178.

Taylor, G. A., 2016. An investigation into the implementation of CYP-IAPT routine outcome measures in their first year of integration into child psychotherapy practice. PhD thesis, University of East London.

The Health Foundation, The King's Fund, 2015. Making change possible: a Transformation Fund for the NHS. The King's Fund.

The Quality Network for Community CAMHS, 2020. Quality Network for Community CAMHS Service Standards. Sixth Edition (2020).

The Quality Network for Community CAMHS, 2016. Quality Network for Community CAMHS Annual Report: Cycle 2015 (January 2015–December 2015).

The Quality Network for Community CAMHS, 2013. Quality Network for Community CAMHS Annual Report: Cycle 7 (2012).

Timimi, S., 2015. Children and Young People's Improving Access to Psychological Therapies: inspiring innovation or more of the same? *BJPsych Bull.* 39, 57–60. https://doi.org/10.1192/pb.bp.114.047118.

Towse, A., Pritchard, C., Devlin, N., 2002. *Cost Effectiveness Thresholds: Economic and ethical issues*. Kings Fund and Office of Health Economics, London.

Tummers, L., Bekkers, V., 2014. Policy Implementation, Street-level Bureaucracy, and the Importance of Discretion. *Public Manag. Rev.* 16, 527–547. https://doi.org/10.1080/14719037.2013.841978.

Varkey, P., Reller, M. K., Resar, R. K., 2007. Basics of Quality Improvement in Health Care. *Mayo Clin. Proc.* 82, 735–739. https://doi.org/10.4065/82.6.735.

Walker, L., Tuffrey, A., Wilson, A., Warner-Gale, F., Street, C., Young Minds, 2014. *Embedding and Sustaining Participation*, in: CYP IAPT 2014 National Conference.

Wolpert, M., Jacob, J., Napoleone, E., Whale, A., Calderon, A., Edbrooke-Childs, J., 2011. *Child-and Parent-reported Outcomes and Experience from Child and Young People's Mental Health Services 2011–2015*. CORC Ltd.

Woods, T., Parsons, S., 2014. *Cross Sector Working: The challenges of difference between health organisation's and the 3rd sector*, in: CYP IAPT 2014 National Conference.

Worrall-Davies, A., 2008. Barriers and Facilitators to Children's and Young People's Views Affecting CAMHS Planning and Delivery. *Child Adolesc. Ment. Health* 13, 16–18. https://doi.org/10.1111/j.1475-3588.2007.00456.x.

Young, D., 2014. Practical Participation–practical hints and tips to help you to involve children and young people in one of the 9 participation priorities, in: CYP IAPT 2014 National Conference.

Chapter 15

Future progress

Hannah Sharp (She/Her) and
Leanne Walker (She/They)

Introduction

This chapter is a call to action. It highlights the key areas for development in the field of participation we wish to see over the coming years. We understand that progress takes time and patience, and that is why we haven't given a timescale for our ambitions here. All we ask, is that everyone who is involved in children and young peoples (CYPs) mental health in some way gives thought to these areas, which are particularly neglected when it comes to participation, and think about how their work can help those areas progress. Participation and involving people with lived experiences in the field, should be everyone's responsibility and it goes without saying, lived-experiences voices should be central to developing this work further.

Measuring Participation

There is a significant need for the development of a measure for participation. Participation is an important, but often under resourced, part of care and service development. Sometimes, in order to ensure the commissioning of more resources for participation, its value needs to be proven; UK National Health Service (NHS) commissioning guidance states that for a service or intervention to be funded it ought to have proven clinical- and cost-effectiveness (NHS Commissioning Board, 2013). While the value of participation can be identified via qualitative means, it is near impossible to prove its clinical- and cost-effectiveness without a quantitative measure. An evidence-base also helps to inform the decisions of policymakers and it is thought to be where good policy comes from (Elliott, 2000). Quantitative evidence forms an important part of creating an evidence-base. Having a strong foundation for participation in policy is necessary because it helps to give weight to its importance when it comes to commissioning. We argue participation can have long-term benefits and impacts, but these are largely uncaptured currently, how can we measure the impact of participation? To individuals, services, organisations, people, groups (etc.), as well as more broadly.

DOI: 10.4324/9781003288800-15

If we are to create a solid evidence-base for participation, we need to understand what the positive and rippling impacts of participation are, beyond just case studies. Using a combined qualitative and quantitative approach allows us to cast a wider net and gain a better national picture of the benefits of participation. It is not to say that anecdotal evidence alone is not of 'proof' or valuable. Qualitative research is incredibly valuable, especially when looking at experiences of participation. What we are proposing is that proving the positive impact of participation in multiple ways, both qualitative and quantitative, short term and long term, helps to solidify our theories and methods of participation.

A further benefit of measuring participation is its role in defining participation. Chapter 1 gave us thoughts on how we can conceptualise participation, and Chapters 3 and 6–13 also talked about what good participation looks like. But this is an ongoing debate and definitions of participation, as well as a consideration of what 'good' participation looks like, has been changing constantly for years. Measuring participation allows us to gain a picture of current thinking around participation. It helps us to focus our discussion on a defined picture of what the 'best' participation looks like. When you have a measure for services to strive towards fulfilling, it focuses the debate on what 'good' participation looks like and helps to limit the variability in this thinking, which comes with a field that is constantly developing. The nature of a developing field as constantly changing raises an interesting question – how do we develop a measure of how good something is when the ideas surrounding what good looks like are constantly changing?

In addition, to measure participation is to see how closely it resembles what the goal for participation is. How do we know if we are doing participation well unless we are seeing how closely what we are currently doing resembles what 'doing well' looks like? Learning about our own practice relating to participation allows us to improve and change how we do it to more closely to resemble the goal. It feeds into the process of learning and development. It informs positive change.

Finally, in the NHS, the idea of 'quality improvement' (QI) is often regarded as the 'gold standard' for service development (NHS England and NHS Improvement, 2022). The QI cycle necessarily involves evaluation. Taking the example of the Plan, Do, Study, Act cycle (PDSA cycle) (ibid.), one cannot 'study' without evaluating the 'doing'. One also cannot 'plan' without knowing where one is at and cannot 'act' without knowing where one is going from. Measuring participation is therefore critical in improving its practice via a QI methodology.

Participation as an Intervention in Its Own Right

Throughout this book we have heard of the benefits of participation to children and young people (CYP) and parents and carers. Some have highlighted the benefits participation has provided to their recovery, yet it is still largely uncaptured by services/within the field. Treating participation as an intervention in its own right allows us to acknowledge these benefits in a young person's care record. This record is their story of the ups and downs of recovery. To omit the role of participation would be to not tell the whole story.

Seeing the value participation has had for some of the CYP throughout this book ought to make us wonder: how can we ensure other young people also benefit from participation? We believe this comes from recognising its therapeutic value and extending participation opportunities to others.

Collaborating with Diverse Communities

At a conference, we once heard someone say that their hope for the future is that we no longer have a need to use the term 'seldom heard voices'. What this means to us, is that participation work engages with all groups and demographic diversity, equitably and everyone's voices are heard, via a variety of different means and creation of spaces. It is important that support structures are in place and by building better and sustainable relationships with different communities, we hope this becomes a reality. We cannot develop services that meet local population need, without local population voice and input.

Lived-experienced Roles

Paying for people's time and the creation of lived experience roles are becoming more common, and we wholeheartedly welcome this. The recognition of the value of lived experience in mental health is a huge change from more recent years. Now, we are beginning to see people's job titles openly share that they have been there themselves. The lived-experience voice brings huge benefits to the field, as highlighted throughout this text. We want to see more lived-experience roles, with better career progression, better support structures and stronger recognition of their value. As a starter, we think it is critical that,

- Lived experienced roles have the right structures in place, including being in a team, with a clear line manager
- Supervision structures, including peer supervision where the unique challenges of working in the lived-experienced field can be discussed
- Career progression and training opportunities exist
- Managers and colleagues understand what it means to employ into lived-experienced roles, with spaces to discuss and reflect with training where required
- Everyone understands each other's roles and responsibilities

- All colleagues have wellness plans in place and workplaces are encouraged to talk about wellbeing.

This Book

Finally, and most importantly, we want this book to become outdated and obsolete. This may seem like a strange goal. Why would editors want their book to no longer be important? What we want, is for this book to be an important part of a journey, but a journey that moves on. We want the journey to move on past the challenges highlighted in this text, to a place where suggestions are implemented, and participation is a fundamental, embedded part of how services function. While it may always serve as a useful guide to come back to, we want the ideas shared throughout to become common thought, such that the book itself doesn't say anything new or 'out there'. We believe this can be achieved, but it requires a commitment towards implementing the ideas and advice throughout the text. Hopefully, we have demonstrated why this is important, but we will leave the final words to a young person, and a parent/carer:

> Participation empowered me to become the person I am today. I want other young people to be able to experience the same and that comes from learning from this book and making change.
>
> Elizabeth (young person)

> This book has shown how life-changing participation can be. Please, consider its lessons and work towards implementing them.
>
> Angela (parent/carer)

References

Elliott, H. 2000. How are policy makers using evidence? Models of research utilisation and local NHS policy making. *Journal of Epidemiology & Community Health*. 54(6), pp.461–468.

NHS Commissioning Board 2013. Commissioning Policy: Ethical framework for priority setting and resource allocation [Online]. Available from: https://www.england.nhs.uk/wp-content/uploads/2013/04/cp-01.pdf.

NHS England and NHS Improvement 2022. Online library of Quality, Service Improvement and Redesign tools. Plan, Do, Study, Act (PDSA) cycles and the model for improvement [Online]. Available from: https://www.england.nhs.uk/wp-content/uploads/2022/01/qsir-pdsa-cycles-model-for-improvement.pdf.

Index

For Product Safety Concerns and Information please contact our EU
representative GPSR@taylorandfrancis.com
Taylor & Francis Verlag GmbH, Kaufingerstraße 24, 80331 München, Germany